TREE OF LIFE

A History of the European School of Osteopathy – and much more…

The First 50 Years

Margery Bloomfield

IndePenPress

Copyright © Margery Bloomfield 2009

All rights reserved

No part of this publication may be reproduced,
stored in a retrieval system, or transmitted
in any form or by any means, without
the prior permission in writing of the publisher,
nor be otherwise circulated in any form of binding or cover other
than that in which it is published and without a similar condition
including this condition being imposed on the subsequent
purchaser.

First published in Great Britain by IndePenPress

All paper used in the printing of this book has been made from
wood grown in managed, sustainable forests.

ISBN13: 978-1-907172-52-6

Printed and bound in the UK
IndePenPress is an imprint of Indepenpress Publishing Limited
25 Eastern Place
Brighton
BN2 1GJ

A catalogue record of this book is available from
the British Library

Cover design by Jacqueline Abromeit

*Dedicated to all who have studied or worked at the E.S.O.
Thank you for enriching my life.*

Contents

Acknowledgements	ii
About the Author	iii
Foreword	v
Introduction	vii
About the Co-Founders	x

Chapter One	A School is Born	1
Chapter Two	Ecole Française d'Ostéopathie (Paris)	6
Chapter Three	Ecole Française d'Ostéopathie (Londres)	16
Chapter Four	The International Federation of Practitioners of Natural Therapeutics (I.F.P.N.T.)	20
Chapter Five	Ecole Européenne d'Ostéopathie (Maidstone)	29
Chapter Six	European School of Osteopathy (Maidstone)	38
Chapter Seven	Society of Osteopaths: The Genesis Osteopathic Foundation	50
Chapter Eight	Politics and Politicians	56
Chapter Nine	European School of Osteopathy	65
Chapter Ten	E.E.O. Developments and International Academic Links	85
Chapter Eleven	European School of Osteopathy	95
Chapter Twelve	Unforgettable Osteopaths and some Unsung Heroes	124
Chapter Thirteen	…and in Conclusion	139

Landmark Dates in the School's History	149
Abbreviations	151
References	153

Acknowledgements

Talking to osteopaths over a number of years about the profession – its past and hopes for its future – persuaded me to take seriously their insistence that I should write the history of the E.S.O. There are too many to mention by name, but I am grateful to them all for those discussions.

Above all I would like to thank John O'Brien. Without his interest and encouragement I doubt that I would have returned to the task after abandoning my first effort.

Once I had got started on my *personal* story there were two dear friends who unfailingly encouraged me. My warmest thanks to Tricia and Mike Armstrong.

Most importantly my sincere thanks to the efficient team at Indepenpress for their support and assistance in seeing this book through production.

M.J.B

About the Author

Margery Bloomfield was co-founder of the European School of Osteopathy with her first husband, the late Tom Dummer, D.O. She was involved with the School from the days when it was in Paris under its original title of Ecole Française d'Ostéopathie. Initially, Margery was administrative director, then principal until her retirement in 1997. She is now a patron of the E.S.O.

Foreword

What an enlightening narrative Margery Bloomfield has written. This is not a tale about one British osteopathic school situated in the Kentish countryside but an account of an osteopathic movement which reached out to continental Europe, long before we were part of the European Economic Community. Nevertheless, the osteopathic stage had been set in the early 1950s when any official connection with its American parent, The American Osteopathic Association (A.O.A.), had been severed and American trained Osteopaths no longer settled in Britain.

This left a void in UK Osteopathy during post-war austerity Britain. Those American trained osteopaths who practised in Britain founded a post-graduate college for medical graduates, London College of Osteopathy (later, the London College of Osteopathic Medicine, L.C.O.M.). Meanwhile, most British osteopathic undergraduate training focussed on the British College of Naturopathy and Osteopathy (B.C.N.O.) and the older, Littlejohn inspired, British School of Osteopahy (B.S.O.). During those formative years the relationship between these establishments and their professional associations was, at best, indifferent and, at worst, distinctly hostile, strong personalities and characters appeared to dominate these groupings. Nonetheless, European osteopathy began to develop its own special modus vivendi assisted by a small but significant group of UK osteopaths. Meanwhile, one of them, Tom Dummer had met and wooed Margery, a public relations consultant..

Their partnership encompassed a close association with Ecole Française d'Ostéopathie (E.F.O.), its transfer to the B.C.N.O. building in North London, under their auspices, and its eventual domicile in Maidstone to be renamed the Ecole Européenne d'Ostéopathie (E.E.O.). With the advent of the four year full time course, the European School of Osteopathy (E.S.O.) emerged during those hectic days. In my opinion through luck or judgement, Tom was able to impart some of the original essence of Andrew Taylor Still's Osteopathy, which had been subsequently misinterpreted, rightly or wrongly, by his followers. Moreover, Margery was there, at all times, soothing bruised egos and organising, and guiding the school through thick and thin, good times and bad, sickness and health. Even when their marriage ended, Margery and Tom maintained their business relationship for the sake of the school's continuance. When Tom retired as E.S.O. principal, Margery continued to control the administrative side, until it dawned on others, she had been de facto principal for decades and appointed her there and then!

By the end of the millennium, she had seen a peripatetic E.F.O. become the E.E.O., and then the E.S.O.. Together with the B.S.O. and the B.C.N.O., the E.S.O. became one of a trio of undergraduate, full-time British colleges recognised by the General Council and Register of Osteopaths (G.C.R.O.) and later the General Osteopathic Council (G.Os.C.). Its graduates gained honours degrees and postgraduate awards validated by associated universities. From such simple Gallic origins, a European movement evolved, Margery was instrumental in its formation and continuance. Along the way she has created a family of graduates and friends who have contributed significantly to their profession's development in the UK, specifically and Europe, in general – this is her story of those eventful times, told with zest.

John O'Brien

Introduction

Osteopathy has been like a river flowing through my life – well, 50 years of it anyway. Writing this book has forced me to reflect on my long association with the osteopathic profession – what has it given me? And what have I been able to give in return?

One thing is sure and certain, it has been an eventful, often bumpy, but always exciting journey. Every step of the way I felt privileged to be part of the unfolding story.

So why did I decide to write this book? Firstly, it was on the suggestion – insistence even – of a number of dear friends in the world of osteopathy who pointed out that I was now the only one left who was there at the beginning when the school was in France, under its original title of Ecole Française d'Ostéopathie. Furthermore, they stressed, I was the only one who knew the *whole* story. What was *not* said, but implied nonetheless, was that I had better get on with it before I fall off my perch. I was beginning to feel duty bound to put pen to paper.

There was another good reason for writing the history. Over the years there has been quite a lot of inaccurate information written about the school – and spoken too no doubt. Sometimes the misinformation, surprisingly, has come from people who should have known better, but the passage of time often distorts the facts. Memory serves some better than others. Perhaps the time had come to put the record straight.

As luck would have it I am blessed with a good memory. Of equal importance, I have been, for as long as I can remember, something of an archivist. As co-founder, administrative director and finally principal of the E.S.O., I have kept my personal copies of the minutes of every board meeting since the school began, as well as copies of the accounts, important reports, correspondence, documents, printed literature, press cuttings – and literally thousands of photographs. Happily, I have been able to draw on these archives for verification of facts and figures.

Half a century is a long time. So much happens in 50 years. The task was daunting and I admit I was a little nervous about what I should put in – and, more importantly, what I should leave out. I confess I am given to a certain naughtiness and the thought crossed my mind that I could write as well an unexpurgated edition. I reasoned that it would sell easily for £100 a copy and raise a lot of money for the school. Prudence however, prevailed and I decided against it. In case there are any graduates or staff members reading this who are wondering whether Margery knew this or that – the answer is yes, probably (not much escaped my notice) but do not worry I am the world's best secret-keeper!

It was about three years ago that I started writing the history, all from memory, working through year by year. By the time I got to the mid '70s the task was becoming tedious. Writing sessions were sporadic – and finally stopped.

I am fortunate in having great friends and a very busy social life. I have loads of hobbies and enjoy fundraising for various local charities. So why was I giving myself a hard time with all this irksome work? It was not as if the school had asked me to write it, nor had it been commissioned by a publisher. The final straw was when, at long last, I read through everything

I had written. It was dry, factually correct, but boring, boring, BORING! I tore up every single page and decided to abandon the project.

In 2008, however, I changed my mind. I received a telephone call from John O'Brien. I had not seen John since the 1990s when he was one of our external examiners for the school. He told me he had retired from practice and was now involved in setting up an osteopathic archive. Would I agree to be interviewed? It was going to be over two days and would be on camera. With some reluctance, I agreed.

It was the preparation for the interview that rekindled my interest, and then talking to John I found my enthusiasm for the task returning. Writing the history of the school was still going to be a considerable challenge, but now I was up for it. Only this time I decided to make it a *personal* story, full of anecdotes and reminiscences.

So here it is. I invite you to look back with me in time. It is my belief that to understand the heartbeat of the European School of Osteopathy, you need to look at its roots and learn something of its history, which is both complex and colourful. I do hope you will enjoy the journey.

M.J.B.
2009

About the Co-Founders

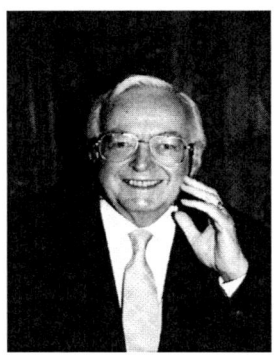

Thomas George Dummer was born in Gerrards Cross, Buckinghamshire, U.K. on the 23rd October 1915. He was an only child. His father was a postman and his mother a seamstress and lady's companion. Tom was rather a sickly child but at an early age he showed musical talent and his parents arranged for him to have piano lessons. At the tender age of four he played on stage in a concert organised by his music teacher.

In his teens he dreamt of becoming a concert pianist but he knew that very few make it to the top and Tom's character was such that he would have been interested only in 'the top'. Although his love of classical music stayed with him all his life, he turned next to jazz. Many were the stories he told of playing in Soho nightclubs – at one point the only white musician in a black jazz band.

For a professional musician it was a disaster when, in 1942, he developed severe pain in his hands. His doctor said it was rheumatism and he would have to learn to live with it. Fortunately, at this moment, he met an American trained Osteopath-Naturopath by the name of Harry Clements, who offered help. During the course of his treatment (which put everything to rights) Tom was becoming ever more interested in natural therapeutics. Eventually he decided to study herbal medicine, whilst continuing his musical career. One of his tutors, Ronald Leisk, was also an osteopath, and it was this contact that inspired Tom to look more deeply into osteopathy. All this was happening during WWII. Tom was a pacifist. By this time he had married twice and had two daughters by his second wife Sarah – Ruth Naomi and Tania Elizabeth.

As well as being a jazz pianist, he was also an accompanist, in particular for Ann Shelton. Decision time came when she was offered an extended tour abroad and she asked Tom if he would go with her. The answer was 'no'. He felt it was time to abandon his musical career and change direction.

Many years later Tom introduced me to Ann Shelton at a Mayfair nightclub where she was singing. Ann had some amusing memories of Tom from that era. For example, she recounted that during breaks in rehearsals, Tom would sit at the piano reading anatomy books and eating grated carrot sandwiches (he was a vegetarian for a few years but finally decided it was not for him).

After the war the British College of Naturopathy was founded and Tom was involved both as a student and, because of his qualification in herbal medicine, as a lecturer as well. He graduated in 1953.

More about Tom anon.

Margery Joan Bloomfield formerly Dummer née Warren – born in Melbourne, Victoria, Australia on the 18th September 1929.

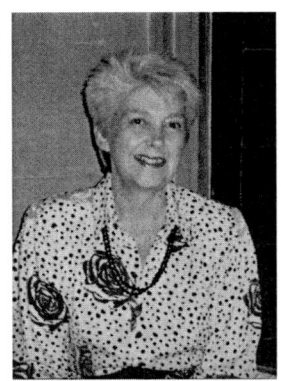

My father was Managing Director of a successful engineering company, which he had founded with a fellow engineer. I had one sister, eight years older. Our parents adored us and each other so my childhood was secure and happy. I loved school, did well and finished up Dux of the school. I was looking forward to going to university to read psychology – but this was not to be. My father became very ill and died. Life turned upside down.

Although I was third generation Australian, oddly enough I never felt I belonged there. From the earliest age I expressed my desire to travel. My dad had travelled in the East for business. I used to sit enthralled with his stories of foreign lands. We had a subscription to the *National Geographic Magazine* and I used to read it cover to cover, preferring it to comics. Following my father's death, I felt like running away – the further the better, but it was not the moment to leave my grieving mother. Instead I abandoned the idea of university, put travel on the back burner, did a business course and then got a job.

By the time I was 21 the travel bug was biting hard. Recognising this my mother gave me the most amazing 21st birthday present – a year long trip around the world with her. It was magical.

I had – indeed I still have – an unquenchable thirst for life. So after some months back in Australia after our travels, my restless spirit began urging me to return to Europe – and back I came in 1953. This time I knew it was for good.

Some more travelling followed including living for a while in Oslo, then Paris before finally settling in London. I guess I was a bit of a vulture for culture at the time, attending classes in psychology, philosophy and art. However, it was high time the gipsy in me made way for some structure and direction in my life. Temporary jobs were all very well but they were not leading anywhere. I liked writing so I took a course in journalism followed by another in public relations. These two courses put me on the road to a career in P.R.

Along the way I was involved in creating London's first Australian restaurant, which was in Beauchamp Place, Knightsbridge where Tom had his bijou flat and practice – but we did not know each other then. I suppose one could say that the hand of fate was creeping ever closer.

Although I had some interesting jobs in advertising and P.R. agencies, I was keen to be more selective about my clients, preferring more artistic and feminine subjects. To this end I started my own P.R. business. As they say 'if opportunity does not knock, build a door!'

Enough about Margery.

Chapter One

A School is Born

'Big oaks from little acorns grow'

PARIS, 1951 – the Ecole Française d'Ostéopathie came into being. The French founder-director was Paul Gény, a state registered physiotherapist with a thirst for finding ever more ways of helping his patients.

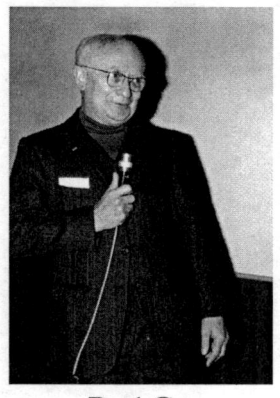

Paul Gény

Our story begins when Paul Gény met an American trained osteopath who was living in Paris – Dr Sterling. Gény was so impressed by all he saw and heard about osteopathy that he determined to study it with the help and guidance of Dr Sterling, since there were no osteopathic schools in France at that early date.

At long last when Gény began to see the results in his practice, he decided that osteopathy had to be shared with colleagues and in 1951 he founded the Ecole Française d'Ostéopathie (E.F.O.) offering a part-time course to state-registered physiotherapists.

In so doing Gény became the 'Father of Osteopathy' in France. It must be remembered that it was illegal at that time for anyone other than a registered medical practitioner to practise osteopathy. Gény reasoned therefore that physiotherapists would be the most likely applicants for his course as they could practise under cover of their physiotherapy diplomas. This proved to be the case.

An interesting coincidence is worthy of mention at this point. In my personal archives I have details of a public auction which took place in the same year as the founding of the E.F.O. – 1951 – of the freehold residence at 104 Tonbridge Road, Maidstone which, many years later, was to become the headquarters of the school. It was at that time known as Bower Hill House and, reading through the details, it must have been an impressive Georgian residence with very large rooms – eight bedrooms, three reception rooms, usual offices, conservatory, a big garden

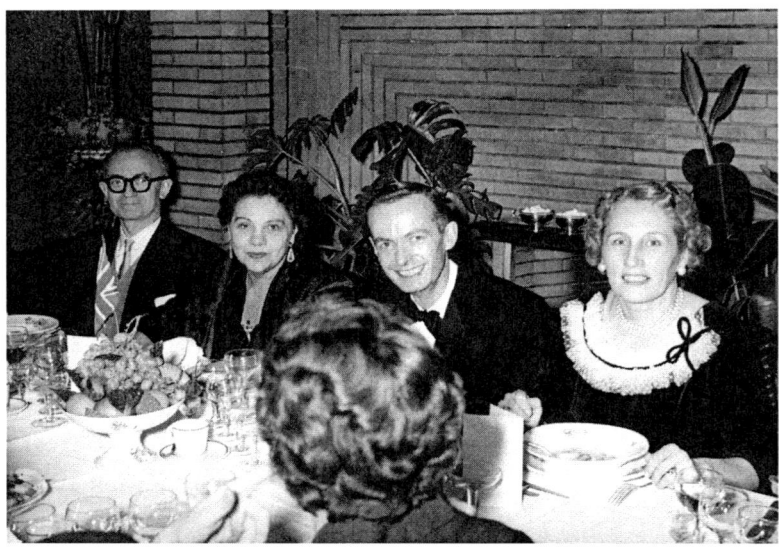

L – R: Paul Gény, Marguerite Maury, Tom Dummer and Mouchette Gény

and outbuildings. It would be fascinating to know what was paid for it.

To return to Paris and Paul Gény, those early days trying to get the school established were tough going. Gradually he gathered a small team of enthusiasts. By 1957 the team included Tom Dummer, an English osteopath, who was introduced to Gény by a mutual friend, Marguerite Maury. Madame Maury was an Austrian born biochemist who lived in Paris and who, incidentally, was the pioneer of aromatherapy.

Tom's command of the French language at that moment in time was not quite up to lecturing standard but the prospect of making regular trips to France was a great incentive for him to make rapid improvement. Rather haltingly at first, Tom Dummer began lecturing at the E.F.O., Paris.

When, you may ask, did Margery appear on the scene? At the end of November, 1959 some mutual friends gave a party to which we were both invited. I recall so clearly that I very nearly decided not to go. It had been a long and difficult day. I was working in public relations and had been out of London covering a story for a client. Returning home at 8pm, the time I should have been arriving at the party, I was exhausted.

The Australian Aboriginals have a word – DADIRRI – which has been described as 'that inner listening from the deep spring that is inside us'. Be that as it may, on the 30th November 1959, a voice from deep within said, with alarming clarity 'Margery forget your tiredness, have a shower, put on your best party dress and GO!' If I had not gone to that party, my life would have been totally different. Amazing, isn't it, how precariously one's future is balanced at times.

So this was the evening I met Tom Dummer and for the first time, heard about osteopathy. Our hosts who were patients of Tom's had mentioned him to me on several prior occasions but always as their naturopath. I rather suspected they were doing a bit of matchmaking that evening. Anyway, we did not need any encouragement, we hit it off immediately soon discovering that we had many similar interests – not least of all our shared love of France. Tom told me he had several French friends he visited from time to time but now, he went on, he was a lecturer at the E.F.O. Paris and was making regular visits. 'What on earth was the E.F.O?' I asked. What indeed!

I then told Tom that my love of France had prompted me to live in Paris for several months learning about all things French, and paying for my frugal 'student life' by teaching English to various nationals who were in Paris doing something similar. (My heart still sings when I recall those crazily wonderful months in Paris.)

Not long after meeting Tom he declared that this was indeed the 'coup de foudre'[1]; in just seven weeks we were married and, guess what, our honeymoon was spent in Paris at a seminar of the E.F.O! As I have been heard to say more than once, I not only married Tom, I married osteopathy as well. (At least one of the marriages lasted!) We were wed in London at Caxton Hall on the 21st January 1960. Tom was 44 and I was 30.

At this juncture I must recount a strange story. Six months or so before meeting Tom, I had left my briefcase on a bus – and did not get it back. It had contained my passport among other items. When I learned that I was going to be honeymooning in Paris, I rang Australia House to request a new passport. I explained that I was going to be wed and would like the new one to be in my married name. Yes, I was told, that would be

---

[1] 'Love at first sight'

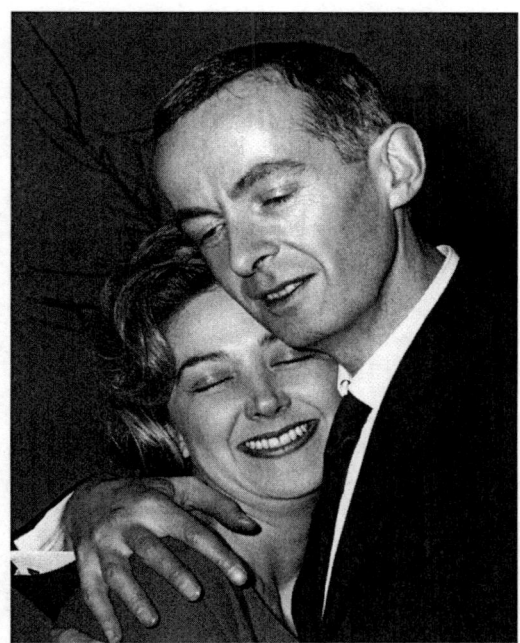

Tom and Margery Dummer on their wedding day

possible, it would be delivered to Caxton Hall and I could collect it after the ceremony. I was then asked for my passport number and date of issue. I had never made a note of these details and did not have the remotest idea. 'We'll have to ring you back' I was told. When the call came through, the voice said '*When* did you say you were getting married?' I repeated '21st January 1960'. Silence, then 'How extraordinary!' he gasped. 'Your passport was due to run out on the 20th January 1960' Wow! Was this one of Jung's meaningful coincidences?

Looking through the photographs that were taken at the reception I am reminded that Parnell Bradbury went with us on our honeymoon, as he too had been invited to lecture at the E.F.O. that week.

Chapter Two

Ecole Française d'Ostéopathie (Paris)

> *'In the centre of difficulty lies opportunity'*
> – Albert Einstein

Our monthly visits to Paris were always enjoyable and action packed. Paul and Mouchette Gény wined and dined us, and looked after our every need. In addition, the students used to vie with one another to entertain us to dinner. Over time our visits to the school became longer, eventually ten days a month, and we began to appreciate our French friends' preoccupation with their livers. 'Une crise de foie' (bilious attack) always solicited enormous sympathy – and rightly so!

In addition to the merrymaking, there was of course lots of work. Lectures and more lectures for Tom who was engaged also in helping Paul rewrite the curriculum. Right from the start I became involved as well, providing secretarial and administration services.

Typing up all Tom's lecture notes taught me a great deal about this new (to me) world of osteopathy – 'a system of manual medicine which lays its main emphasis on the structural and mechanical problems of the body'. I learned that the theory of osteopathy was set out in 1874 by an American physician, Andrew Taylor Still. Through his clinical experience as a doctor, Still discovered the vital relationship between the structure (anatomy) and functions of the human organism (physiology). Although the body is a self-healing unit, it often needs some help from the osteopath who will hunt the cause of the problem before treating.

I learned also that Dr Still went on to establish the first college of osteopathic medicine at Kirksville, Missouri, U.S.A. which was charted in 1892.

Two students of Still had a great influence on the development of osteopathy. Dr J. Martin Littlejohn contributed greatly to the physiological understanding of osteopathic medicine. Dr William Garner Sutherland's contribution was in the understanding of the cranial mechanism. I took to the principles of naturopathy with equal enthusiasm. All this new knowledge made such sense to me, I was hooked – and have remained so.

The E.F.O.'s premises were on the Boulevard St. Germain on the Left Bank. We stayed nearby, always at the same hotel – small, unpretentious and very French. Before we were married, on his visits to Paris Tom had stayed in a small flat on the Île St. Louis belonging to Marguerite Maury and, during the same periods, she borrowed his bijou flat in Beauchamp Place, Knightsbridge. This gave her a London base at which she could see clients, thereby introducing aromatherapy to the U.K. In no time Marguerite was in such demand that she decided to relocate to London where she set up her own aromatherapy clinic. She did not just look after the beauty of the rich and famous, Marguerite Maury did some remarkable work with skin problems and, especially impressive, was her ability to minimize scars following accidents. I had the good fortune to have some memorable facials from her. I arrived one day at her clinic and she announced that she wanted me to model for an article that was being written about her work – the photographer was already set up and waiting. The idea was to take before and after photographs. For this particular aspect of her work she wanted to demonstrate what could be achieved using just her hands, no essential oils or creams on this occasion. When I looked in the mirror following the treatment, I could hardly believe the difference. She had the most amazing hands.

It was important to give the French students as broad an osteopathic training as possible. To this end Tom rallied many English colleagues to join the E.F.O. faculty. Names that spring to mind include John Wernham, Brian Youngs, Parnell Bradbury, Dr Dudley Tee, Colin Winer, Denis Brookes. There was a willingness by one and all to lecture in Paris, as it was such an enjoyable experience.

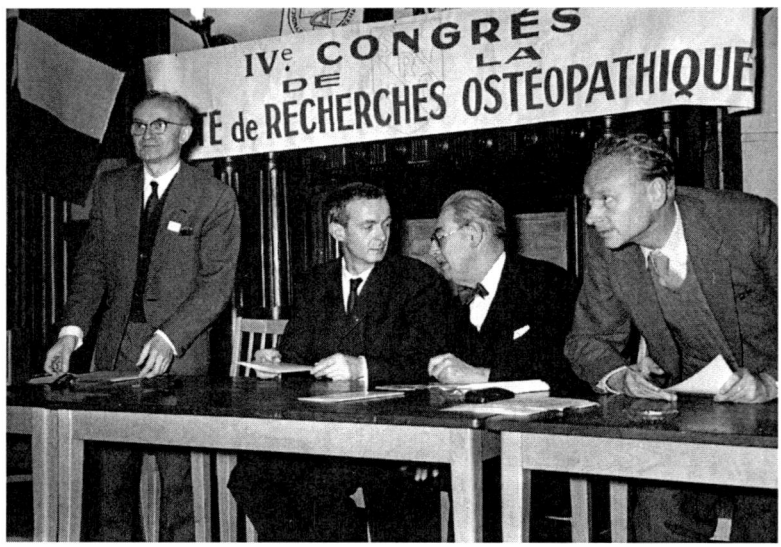

Fourth congress of the S.R.O.
L – R: Paul Gény, Tom Dummer, Phillip Knaggs and Parnell Bradbury

Paul Gény played his part too in forging links with the osteopathic profession in the U.K. In addition to founding the E.F.O. he started as well the S.R.O. – Société de Recherches Ostéopathiques, and English colleagues were invited to participate in the conferences. The Entente Cordiale was reinforced by a memorable Anglo-French conference of the S.R.O. held in the U.K. in November 1961. My archives include a signed menu from that event.

Paul made many visits to London, always dropping in at the British College of Naturopathy. He also attended the bi-annual conferences of the association, thereby cementing friendships with English colleagues. Eventually, Paul took the External D.O. of the college.

When I was first involved with the profession I recall how confused I was with all the initials of organisations and qualifications in the field of natural therapeutics, and people would talk in initials too. For those who need it, I have added a list of abbreviations at the back of this book. However, before continuing with our story I think a word of explanation is needed regarding the various titles of the naturopathic college and association. First of all, for the uninitiated, naturopathy is the professional practice of those therapies based upon the Nature Cure concept – of which more a little later. A college for the study of naturopathy had started in 1936, but the war interrupted activities and it had to close. Then on the initiative of naturopath, Stanley Lief, the British College of Naturopathy (B.C.N.) came into being in 1949, along with the British Naturopathic Association (B.N.A.) which was formerly the Nature Cure Association of Great Britain and Ireland. In 1961 a decision was taken to incorporate the word osteopathy into the title of both organisations making them – British College of Naturopathy and Osteopathy (B.C.N.O.) and British

Naturopathic and Osteopathic Association (B.N.O.A.). Today the college is called British College of Osteopathic Medicine and referred to as B.com.

Returning to that grand pioneer Stanley Lief, it is interesting to reflect on his many achievements. For example, he started Champneys as a Nature Cure resort. Today of course it is a very different place but the name lingers on. Stanley was also the founder and editor of the magazine *Health for All* – of which I have a copy dated June 1956 (what a squirrel I am) and in it is an article by Thomas G. Dummer entitled *Radiesthesia – Has it a place in Nature Cure Practice.* I recall with a smile Stanley's wife Stella Lief, who was Hon. Secretary of the B.C.N. She was a huge enthusiast for naturopathy and when one day a patient died, Stella declared 'Well, yes, but she died having the right treatment'. That story was often repeated.

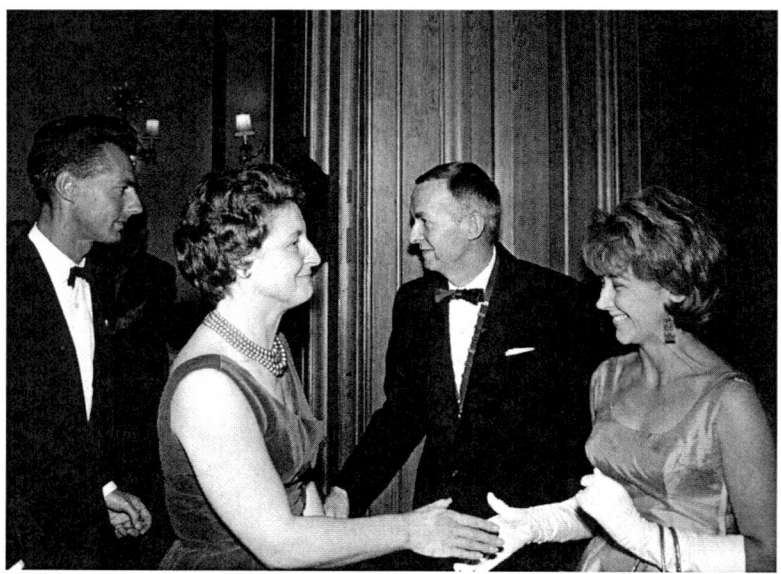

Tom – President of the B.N.O.A. – 1961
With Margery, greeting guests

Tom was elected twice as president of the B.N.O.A in the early part of the 1960s. During this period I offered public relations services to the B.N.O.A in an honorary capacity. I have some interesting documents in my archives. One worthy of mention is the 1963 report of a commission set up to standardize naturopathic nomenclature. Oh, how they argued! There were those who saw naturopathy as embracing dietetics, fasting, natural hygiene, hydrotherapy, education in Nature Cure philosophy and structural adjustments – by such methods as osteopathic, chiropractic and neuromuscular techniques, remedial exercises and postural re-education. Then there were others who wanted to include, in addition to the foregoing, medical herbalism, homoeopathy, therapeutic biochemistry etc. providing of course the practitioners concerned were qualified in these specialised therapies. The big argument however, raged around osteopathy. There were those in the Nature Cure movement who viewed osteopathy as *a part of* naturopathy. Such a minor

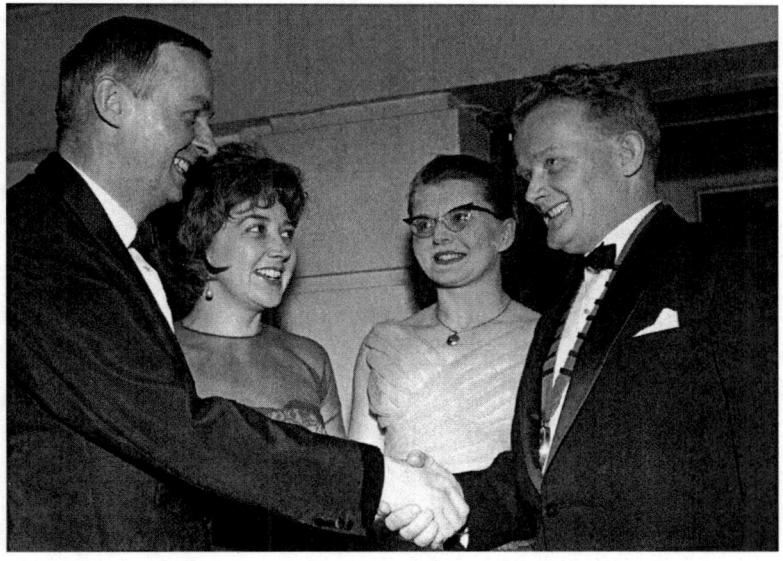

Tom handing over to new President Albert Rumfitt

role was totally unacceptable to practitioners who knew osteopathy to be a vast subject worthy of an independent identity. Recalling all those heated debates, it is interesting to ponder that the same naturopathic college is now called British College of Osteopathic Medicine.

One of my tasks when acting as Hon. P.R.O. was to keep an eye out

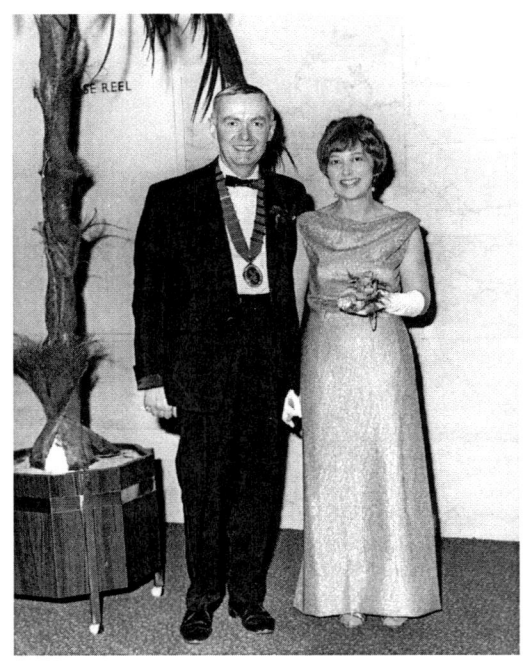

Tom and Margery – 1965 presidency of B.N.O.A.

for any literature or statements in the press, which suggested that *only* those who were members of the General Council and Register of Osteopaths (G.C. and R.O.) were competent to practise osteopathy. The day came when the British School of Osteopathy (at the time the only school recognised by the G.C. and R.O. apart from the doctor osteopaths' group) issued a leaflet which caused hackles to rise throughout the membership of the B.N.O.A. I made contact with the association's solicitors, and the outcome was most satisfactory. The offending leaflet was withdrawn, coupled with an assurance that any future publication by them would be entirely factual. More importantly, through their solicitors they also stated that they did not wish to do anything that might encourage dissension within the profession. This occurred in 1963. In spite of these intermittent skirmishes, there were signs of slight improvement in relations with registered osteopaths. For example there was a slow trickle of G.C. and R.O. members into membership of the B.N.O.A. and a coming together of osteopaths from both organisations at events organised by John Wernham in Maidstone.

During this period I had a press cutting service whereby any mention of naturopathy or osteopathy in the press would be sent to me. I had only one smallish box of cuttings until… the scandal of the century, when all of a sudden I had press cuttings piled heavens high. This was 'The Profumo Affair' at the centre of which was the society osteopath, Dr Stephen Ward. For those who do not know about this real life story, let me tell you it involved everything that sells newspapers – politics, sex, lies, spies, drugs, call girls, people in high society and, finally, Stephen Ward's suicide.

Ward died on 3rd August 1963 and by then, with the vast amount of media coverage that had ensued, there was nobody left in the U.K. who did not know what an osteopath was. Whatever Ward may or may not have been, I understand from those who knew him that he was a very good osteopath. He was also a talented artist and I was delighted to have a couple of his sketches hanging on the wall in my office at the school, left to us by Teddy Hall who had been the subject of some of Ward's drawings.

The call girl in the Profumo Affair was Christine Keeler. When Tom and I moved the practice from Chelsea to Bingham Place near Baker Street, we discovered that Christine Keeler lived in the vicinity and what is more her telephone number was similar to ours. One day we were busy in the practice when the telephone rang and a voice said 'May I speak to Christine Keeler'. I thought straight away it was a friend of ours who always said something silly when I answered the 'phone, so I went along with 'the joke' and replied in my sexiest voice 'Christine is not in but *I'm* here'. 'And who are you?' I replied, 'You had better come round and find out'. Eagerly he agreed and said he would be there in half an hour. Suddenly I realised the call was for real!

By this time Paul Gény was coming over to London for a few days each month to work with Tom in the practice offering acupuncture, which Paul had studied under Dr Jacques Lavier. Their two individual treatment approaches complemented each other to the great benefit of many selected patients. An acquaintance of ours, who was a journalist, heard about Gény's monthly visits and asked if he could write an article about him. When it appeared in a high circulation woman's magazine, our practice telephone never stopped ringing. Acupuncture had arrived in the U.K!

Back in Paris however things were getting more and more difficult for Paul. Paradoxically, it was not illegal to *teach* osteopathy – indeed in January 1964 the E.F.O. was recognised by l'Académie de Paris – but it was illegal to practise it, if you were not a registered medical practitioner. The authorities therefore could not close down the school but what they could do – and did relentlessly – was fine Paul Gény for the illegal practice of medicine.

Tom and I decided to mount a campaign in support of Paul's predicament. We circularized the osteopathic profession in the U.K. urging colleagues to send letters of protest to Général de Gaulle and the Ministre de la Santé. There was a great response but it was all to no avail. It should be remembered that in those early days there was no statutory recognition of osteopaths in the U.K. either, but all practised legally under Common Law.

Eventually the number of fines Gény received became an impossible financial burden for him to carry. Although he had lost the battle he was not willing to accept defeat. Instead he asked us if we could run the E.F.O. from England! It sounded crazy but we were eager to help. Here we were agreeing to take on the training of French students in a country that was not *their* own, in a language that was not *our* own and, when qualified, they would be practising something that was against the law anyway! Were we mad or what! The thing is we thought we would be completing the education of those students who had started their studies in Paris – and that would be the end of it. Little did we think that the school would take off in the way that it did.

CHAPTER THREE

Ecole Française d'Ostéopathie (Londres)

> *'Where nothing is sure, everything is possible'*
> – Margaret Drabble

THE FIRST TASK was to find accommodation for the school. Tom approached the B.C.N.O. They agreed to offer their Hampstead premises during weekends and holiday periods. This was a great solution.

Of all the enrolled students in Paris, in the end only 16 elected to cross the Channel in order to complete their studies in London. Although Paul Gény remained a member of faculty, he passed the mantle of principal of the E.F.O. (Londres) to Tom, whilst my task was to deal with the administration and finances. On the subject of finance, there was none! All we had inherited were 16 students – no money, no equipment, no books, no skeletons – in or out of the cupboard, NOTHING. On the day the E.F.O. (Londres) opened its doors, the thought for the day on my desk calendar read: 'Nothing great was ever achieved without enthusiasm'. If there was one thing we were not lacking it was enthusiasm, we had bags of it and were determined to make this work.

We came to an agreement with the B.C.N.O. whereby the E.F.O. became a part of their registered charity, in effect the French postgraduate department of the B.C.N.O. The fees from the students would be paid directly into the B.C.N.O.'s bank account and one third of the total income would be retained by them in lieu of rent, with one third to cover lecturers' fees and the final third to pay for everything else. It felt as if someone had given us a lump of modelling clay with the instruction to go away and create a school. Quite a challenge!

The first seminar began on 13th December 1965. Although we were functioning now as a part of the B.C.N.O., academically we remained independent. The move to London had been arranged at top speed and the only lecturers available were Tom Dummer and Paul Gény. One of so many problems we faced was that of language, so few English osteopaths being French-speaking. A bilingual friend, Graham Clarke, agreed to help us with written material. For the second seminar we obtained the services of a professional English/French interpreter through an agency. After less than a day, she fled never to return. It was understandable; she had no knowledge of osteopathy and not much medical terminology either, so it was a hopeless task. Then we met Martine who was French, living in London and a student at the B.C.N.O. Perfect! She remained our official interpreter for many years. When Martine Faure-Alderson graduated from the B.C.N.O., she also came to work with us in the practice and later lectured in the school as well.

Soon we were gathering an impressive faculty, some of whom had lectured previously at the E.F.O. (Paris). For the next seminar we had Parnell Bradbury, Colin Winer and Brian Youngs. Then in 1966 we met Peter Blagrave and he in turn introduced us to Barrie Savory – and many more followed. The faculty list was beginning to look like the 'Who's Who' in osteopathy. This

French school in exile caught the imagination and seemed to bring out the rebel in everyone whilst, in France, news of the E.F.O. (Londres) went around the physiotherapy profession like wildfire. To our surprise applications to join the school began to pour in and by the late 1960s we had a two-year waiting list. Having outgrown the space available to us in London, we asked John Wernham if we could have some overflow seminars at his osteopathic clinic in Kent. An unequivocal 'yes' was his reply. This was the school's first contact with Maidstone.

With increased student numbers came increased income for the B.C.N.O. The bursar/treasurer H. Bagnall Goodwin, often expressed satisfaction that 'the French', (as he always referred to the E.F.O.) were keeping the B.C.N.O. out of the red. Of course it was not just 'the French' anymore. By 1970 we had many Belgian students and then French-speaking Spanish, Swiss and Portuguese. Eventually a decision was taken to change the name of the school, more appropriately, to Ecole Européenne d'Ostéopathie. I have in my files the document confirming that decision. It was dated 1st April 1971, to operate from the new academic year 1971–72 and signed by Paul Gény and Tom Dummer.

Concurrent with the success of the school came rumblings within the B.C.N.O. and the B.N.O.A. Those who were around at the time may well have their own interpretation of events, but I am adhering to the facts backed up by my archive material. Concern was expressed that the E.F.O. had become a school within a school. There were fears that it might even overtake the B.C.N.O. in importance. Talk also of the tail wagging the dog. I heard an opinion expressed that it was the French cigarette-smoking habit that caused the rift. I do not doubt it would have been frowned upon, and rightly so, but the reason for the split was much more complicated. To add to the above mix, there was also the vexed question of the B.C.N.O. refusing to join the International Federation of Practitioners of Natural Therapeutics – of which more in the next chapter.

Marie Curie is quoted as saying 'Nothing in life is to be feared. It is to be understood'. There were many strong personalities around at the time – on all sides – and any hope of 'understanding' went out the window. The E.F.O. was made to feel less and less welcome. The split from the B.C.N.O. was nigh. We decided to discuss the situation with John Wernham.

Chapter Four

The International Federation of Practitioners of Natural Therapeutics (I.F.P.N.T.)

> *'Inside every large problem is a small problem struggling to get out'*

EARLY IN THE 1960s there was growing concern about the possible implications of the Treaty of Rome as and when Great Britain joined the Common Market. In May 1962 the Deutsche Heilpraktikeschaft (D.H.), which was the organisation representing natural therapy practitioners in Western Germany, issued an invitation to attend an informal meeting in Essen at the time of their annual congress, to discuss these issues. Delegates from Great Britain, France and Holland met under the chairmanship of Josef Angerer, then president of the D.H. After long discussion it was unanimously agreed that a committee be set up with the title 'International Committee for Natural Therapeutics' and Tom Dummer was elected general secretary. The I.C.N.T.'s task was to prepare for the founding of an international organisation to represent non-medically registered bona fide practitioners of all the natural therapies worldwide.

Much work was involved contacting organisations throughout Europe and beyond. Finally, on February 18th 1965

The International Federation of Practitioners of Natural Therapeutics was incorporated as a non-profit making company limited by guarantee, in pursuance of the Companies Act, 1948. Later it was registered also under the Charities Act. Tom was elected Hon. Secretary General, Margery Assistant Hon. Secretary General, Brian Youngs Hon. Treasurer and the President was to be by rotation.

The aims and objects of the new company are too numerous to reproduce here. In summary, the I.F.P.N.T. stood for the advancement of natural therapeutics on every level leading to the progressive elevation of education and practice standards ensuring an ethical, efficient, alternative health service in all countries associated with the movement. In addition it aimed to protect the public as far as ever possible from the unqualified practitioner and, ultimately, to ensure freedom of choice in medical care for every individual.

So, not much to do! However it was fascinating work and we loved every minute of it. We met some very interesting people and did a lot of travelling in the process. The I.F.P.N.T. could well provide the material for a book all on its own.

There are certain aspects of the work we did which are worth relating here. For example we spent a lot of effort trying to stamp out 'diploma mills'. These were operated by unscrupulous individuals who *sold* qualifications in osteopathy, naturopathy, herbal medicine – in fact anything you wanted. The main targets for these reprehensible activities were the Third World countries. The diplomas, in whichever discipline, were usually large with lots of gold and flourishing signatures to make them look 'impressive' on the walls of the quack's consulting rooms. Oh, those poor unsuspecting patients. In unregulated professions of course, this sort of thing can happen. Over time we built up a vast amount of evidence and duly reported our findings. The result was that Interpol arrived one day and took away all our files for photocopying. They seemed to be impressed by all the material we had gathered.

Within the E.E.C. countries at that time there was an incongruous legal situation for all non-medically registered practitioners of natural therapeutics. Western Germany was the only country to have statutory regulation (introduced, incidentally, by Hitler). In Great Britain and the Republic of Ireland practitioners were in a unique position in that they practised freely under Common Law. In the Netherlands, at the time, it was illegal but tolerated; in Denmark allowed but with considerable restrictions imposed by Quackery Acts. In France, as already explained, it was illegal. In Belgium it was even worse as practitioners could be imprisoned for the illegal practice of medicine, even any kind of meeting of practitioners was against the law. It was illegal also in Italy and Spain. Interestingly, it was the countries where Napoleonic law formed the basis of their judicial systems that were the most repressive.

Speaking of Belgium, I recall a dramatic sequence of events which occurred in 1973 when the practices of 28 chiropractors were visited by the police serving notice for the illegal practice of medicine. In effect they were closing them down, with the warning that should there be a 'next time' it would be a gaol sentence. In a number of instances, we were told, the policeman concerned was a patient, so it was a case of entering by the front door to serve the summons for closure, and then going around to the back door to keep an appointment for treatment. How crazy!

As we researched the situation around the world it became clear that the legal status of practitioners differed from one country to another and even from state to state within the same country. For example in Australia at that time, only the state of Western Australia had statutory recognition and only for chiropractic, whilst in Canada only some of the provinces had laws for osteopathy, chiropractic and naturopathy. In Switzerland only one Canton, Appenzell, permitted the practice of natural therapeutics, although in the country as a whole chiropractic had achieved statutory recognition.

By contrast, in India, natural therapies were inherent in the Indian tradition and had become an intrinsic part of village life, being closely associated with Ghandian ideals. Early in 1973 we made our second visit to India where we had many contacts, which meant that we had the good fortune to be able to stay with various families, rather than in hotels. We also received wonderful hospitality from the All India Nature Cure Federation, which was a member of the I.F.P.N.T. Indeed we were accorded V.I.P. status. We were invited to tea with the President of India (Desai was a devotee of nature cure). Then at a public meeting in Delhi, presided over by the Minister of Health, Tom was asked to speak on behalf of the I.F.P.N.T. Following this the Government of India requested the International Federation to advise their department of health on all aspects of natural therapeutics as they may pertain to India.

We stayed with another I.F.P.N.T. member, the Arogya Mandir Nature Cure Home in Gorakphur. It was intensely interesting to see at first hand how it operated and observe the range of treatments they offered. Whilst there, our host kindly arranged for us to be taken on a pilgrimage tour of the Buddhist sites. This was an unforgettable experience for both of us.

We also had some visits to hospitals and clinics. Particularly memorable, although heartbreaking, was the Leprosy Centre.

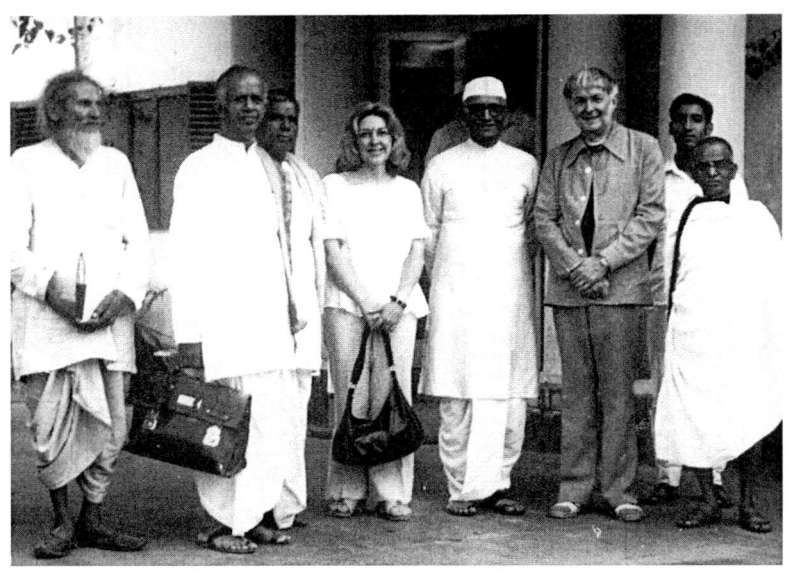

Tom and Margery meeting with the President of India

Then there was the hospital on four floors with each floor devoted to a different approach to medical care – orthodox, homoeopathic, ayurvedic, and naturopathic.

I enjoyed too visiting a Ghandian village and seeing all the measures they had developed to make themselves self-sufficient. Decentralisation and the redevelopment of village community life were central to the Ghandian ideals. I was asked to plant a tree to mark the occasion of our visit – which brings to mind another tree-planting episode. When I retired in 1997, one of my leaving presents was a Lebanese cedar tree which was planted with much ceremony in the grounds of Boxley House. Unfortunately, nobody looked after it and it died – even the touchingly worded brass plate 'disappeared'. I hope my tree in India fared better.

Back in 1965, the I.F.P.N.T. had its first meeting in Brussels with a high ranking official of the E.E.C. Commission, a

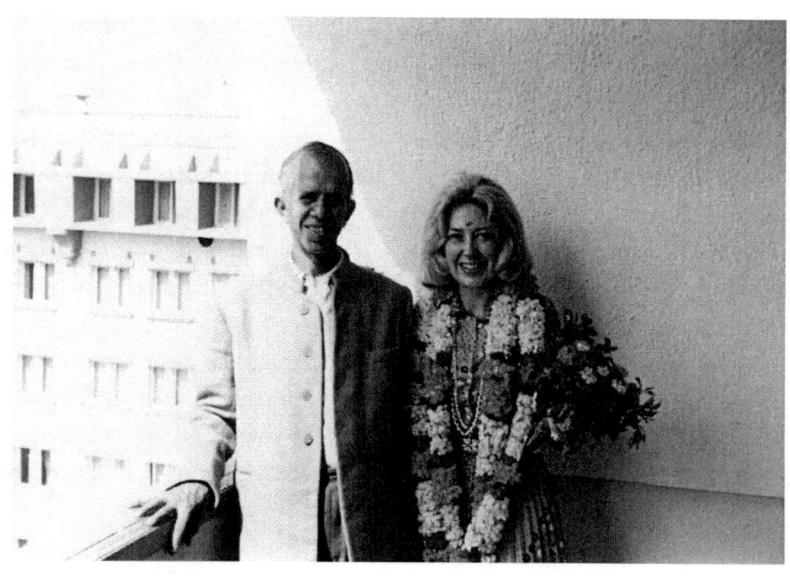

Margery – bedecked with flowers – a daily occurence and our host from the All India Nature Cure Federation

Monsieur J.P de Crayencour. The advice we received then and at subsequent meetings was always along similar lines, and confirmed repeatedly by our parliamentary lobby and our international law consultant. In essence, if we were to survive in the Common Market then the I.F.P.N.T.'s main thrust had to be standardisation and progressive raising of educational standards, and unity of all bona fide practitioners of natural therapies. Fragmented professions, we were told again and again, would not be listened to by anyone. 'Put your house in order' was the message. Unity, for sure, was the most challenging item on the agenda. There was so much infighting, so many big personalities, and so many clashes within organisations and within the individual professions – and it was happening nationally and internationally. The late Clem Middleton D.O. famously coined the collective noun 'a difference of osteopaths' – and so it was throughout natural therapeutics. It seemed to be something that went with the territory.

Nobody did more for unity than Tom Dummer and yet he, too, was given to having rows with colleagues throughout his life. As a friend of his once said to me, with restrained affection, 'Scorpios are great builders – *and* – destroyers. Beware of the sting in his tail'. One rift that I have never forgotten was when Tom fell out with Paul Gény over an incident in an I.F.P.N.T. meeting. To be frank, Tom was being insensitive and rather disloyal and Paul was being incredibly stubborn. The shutters went up on both sides of the Channel, causing a lot of ripples on the water. Ange Castejon, fearing their disagreement would have a harmful effect on the school, stepped in and invited all interested parties to his home in Lyon. After a glass or three, and some frank speaking, peace returned (although I felt, with sadness, that their relationship never recovered completely).

When I reflect on those early days, it is no wonder the movement had a reputation for being 'prickly'. There was so much to fight against – and for. Anyone entering a branch of natural therapeutics was (a) at variance with the orthodox system of medicine, (b) outside the establishment and (c) in many countries, illegal as well. Consequently, natural therapeutics attracted individualists, independently minded people usually with a streak of rebellion running through their veins, and a lot of strongly held opinions. Nevertheless, whatever differences of opinion there were, we just had to work through them with the ultimate objective of presenting a united front both to governments and the E.E.C. Commission. This was essential if statutory recognition was ever to be achieved.

On the home front there were two major problems. Through the Federation's contacts in Brussels, we were advised that the West German Heilpraktiker Schools should get together with the B.C.N.O. as the largest full-time natural therapeutics training college in Great Britain in order to co-ordinate their teaching standards. As Western Germany was the only European country to have statutory regulation, it followed that their standards would perforce be accepted as the criterion for all the other countries. However, in Great Britain, although there was no statutory regulation at that time, it was not illegal. In 1973 when Great Britain became a full member of the E.E.C., the advice we had received was strengthened further. The problem was that the B.C.N.O. refused to join the I.F.P.N.T., even though the B.N.O.A. passed a resolution at its A.G.M. in May 1973 that the B.C.N.O. should become an associate member. The board of governors of the college dug their heels in and decided, without dissent, that membership of the I.F.P.N.T. 'was not in the best interests of the B.C.N.O.' Their decision was conveyed to the members of the B.N.O.A. at an extraordinary general meeting held in October 1973, the result of which was a further resolution from the floor expressing no confidence in the board of governors. This was refuted by the board who claimed that the B.C.N.O. standards were substantially higher than that operating in other countries; therefore they did not wish to be identified with groups whose standards did not match their own. How they could be so convinced of this when they had refused to have any dialogue, even with the statutorily regulated D.H. schools, remained a mystery. Their stance showed that they were completely missing the point of all the work that was being done by the I.F.P.N.T.

This 'holier than thou' attitude existed in other areas as well. The General Council and Register of Osteopaths (G.C. and R.O.) came into being in 1936 with the laudable aim of becoming fully representative of the osteopathic profession in Great Britain. The majority of its membership consisted of graduates from the British School of Osteopathy (B.S.O.) plus some others who were admitted by external examination under article 11 of the constitution of the G.C. and R.O. This form of entry was closed in 1952; after that date only graduates of the B.S.O. or doctor osteopaths were eligible for membership.

As time went on, this rigid policy of exclusivity became increasingly unacceptable to the other osteopathic groups and schools. The G.C. and R.O. claimed to be *the* authority for deciding the competence of osteopaths. In reality *all* osteopaths, regardless of their affiliations, practised under Common Law. The G.C and R.O. was of course a voluntary register as were the other osteopathic organisations' registers of members.

Unhappily, the G.C. and R.O. was weakening the move towards unity of the osteopathic profession. Things had to change – and they did, as will be seen later.

CHAPTER FIVE

Ecole Européenne d'Ostéopathie (Maidstone)

> *'Don't be afraid to take a big step if one is indicated,
> you can't cross a chasm in two small jumps'*
> – David Lloyd George

JOHN WERNHAM WAS aware already of the difficulties we had been experiencing at the B.C.N.O. Without hesitation he agreed that the school could function entirely from his premises in Maidstone. Thus, in 1971, the newly named Ecole Européenne d'Ostéopathie (E.E.O.) relocated to Kent. I must emphasize that it was only the name that changed – the students, faculty, principal and 'staff' (all one of me) were the same, as was the curriculum.

Having left behind for the B.C.N.O. whatever modest sum was over, we started again, this time as a part of John Wernham's registered charity.

Concurrent with all the developments, a unique and timely opportunity presented itself. The house adjoining John's clinic came on the market. 'Only a pessimist would complain about the noise, when opportunity knocks.' Everything felt so positive in 1971 – cooperation and optimism ruled! Without delay the Maidstone Osteopathic Clinic (M.O.C.) bought No. 28 Tonbridge Road. The stars were smiling down on us!

The E.E.O. was formally incorporated into the M.O.C. as the educational and research unit of the charity and Tom was appointed as its principal. This is an opportune moment to correct something I have seen in print. John Wernham was *never* principal of the school, he was the director of the clinic, a member of faculty and our landlord.

Prior to these events Tom and I had been members of the M.O.C. committee. Now John asked me if I would accept the appointment of secretary/treasurer of the clinic committee. My workload was already huge but I wanted to help and accepted.

With our newly named and newly located school, we needed new letterheads and an emblem, ideally a design that would encompass osteopathy and the spirit. We sat around the kitchen table discussing the possibilities and sketching ideas for logos.

It was Tom who came up with the design and the following is an extract from an article he wrote on 'the esoteric symbolism of the E.E.O. logo' which later of course became the E.S.O. logo as well:-

'The origins of the symbolism expressed in the E.S.O. logo go back into antiquity and belong to the esoteric tradition. It was felt that the E.S.O. logo should reflect both the spiritual as well as the material basis of osteopathy, i.e. in the same tradition of STILL himself, spiritual as well as scientific. I found my inspiration in *The Secret Doctrine* by Madame Blavatsky a controversial figure in the early days of Theosophy.

First of all the logo is composed of two triangles. Triangular form expresses balance and relativity and thus wholeness. This is evident in the Littlejohn system of body mechanics and dynamics, where the interaction of gravitational forces form so-called triangles of force and relate to each other in dynamic equilibrium. This is in a physical-mechanical sense.

On the physio-chemical level the three sided or three dimensional aspects are Anabolism, Catabolism and Metabolism.

On the spiritual and esoteric levels the triangle expresses the indivisibility of the Triad – in Christianity the Holy Trinity, in Hinduism based on the teachings of the Vedas – Brahma, Vishnu and Siva, in Buddhism the Trikaya – the Three Bodies of Buddha and in the Quabbala symbolic triangles are found for example in the symbol of Binah. The pyramids of ancient Egypt consist of three triangles in apposition on a triangular base, a very powerful stratagem for concentrating energy – capable in fact of mummification. Pyramids are also found in Mexico and it is claimed – on the Moon and Mars.

Returning to the E.S.O. logo, accompanying the two triangles is the quaternary which is below the upper triangle and closer to earth, whereas the inner triangle is higher and closer to heaven. Together the inner triangle and the quaternary form the symbol of septenary "man", who has seven dimensions, seven layers of existence and seven aspects of being, in all the Totality.

I put the Atlas vertebra in the middle of the quaternary since it is at the summit of the spinal column where it ultimately supports the head. Symbolically in the same way Atlas in Greek mythology, supported the world on his shoulders. Likewise it is the focal point of all the different physical qualities represented in the E.S.O. triangle generally.

The placing of the "O" (Osteopathy) from E.S.O./E.E.O. in the middle of the inner triangle has further significance, since it connotes the spiritual dimension, whereas E and S or E and E placed next to the quaternary represent the physical dimension.

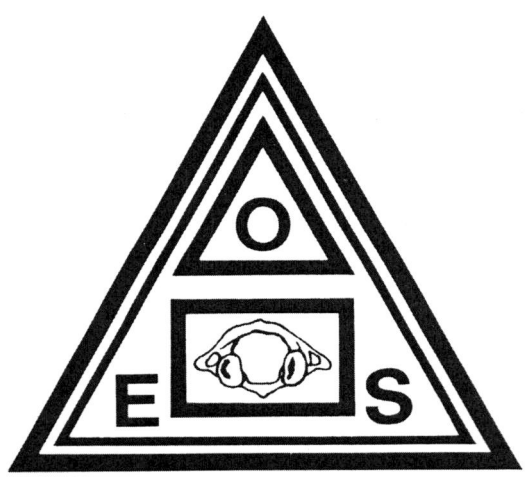

A triangle and quaternary together is the symbol of Septenary Man (Homosapiens). The number six is regarded as the emblem of the physical nature i.e. the six dimensions of all physical bodies – the length (height) and breadth (width), the two lines of thickness, the top and the bottom (crown of head and soles of feet) analogous in a spatial sense to the four cardinal points – N, S, E and W and the Zenith and the Nadir. These six dimensions (the Senary) equal the physical attributes. Add one more dimension – the immortal consciousness or soul and this makes seven, representing the Septenary – the Totality.'

The article continues but I think that is quite enough of the logo – except to say, nearly 30 years later, when Renzo Molinari had taken over as principal, he introduced a new logo with the design help of Colin Wallis. The main elements of our original logo were still present but less esoteric: the new design gave an up-to-date image. I liked it very much but I must admit to a slight pang of sadness to see the old one disappear.

Returning to the E.E.O. course, initially it was of five years duration of postgraduate studies. Subsequently we increased it to six years, which was a long time to be following a course in another country. It called for considerable sacrifices on the part of the students for whom, in all the circumstances, I had the greatest admiration. The part-time course was not in any sense an easy option; they had a vast amount of material to get through.

By the time we moved to Maidstone, the English faculty had been joined by several French lecturers, in particular Ange Castejon who later was to play a big part in the development of the E.E.O.

Our French speaking students were appreciative of studying at the M.O.C. as they were ever mindful of the importance of apostolic succession: A.T. Still, Founder of Osteopathy, had taught J. Martin Littlejohn who later taught John Wernham. The students sometimes referred to the apostolic succession as Still – Littlejohn – and Big John.

So many anecdotes flood back when I remember those early days of the E.E.O. The students seemed to regard me as the source of all information. I was asked constantly where they could shop in their lunch breaks for this or that. Marks & Spencer was top favourite and they would come back laden with bags. Electrical goods, which were then much cheaper here, were another favourite whilst some favoured rummaging in Mrs Turk's antique shop. Between hotel/b&b accommodation, restaurants, pubs and shopping, the E.E.O. did a lot for the economy of Maidstone.

There were requests for my help in more personal areas as well. For example, 'Where can I buy "le Baby Pill"?' or on one occasion 'can you arrange for me to have a vasectomy in my lunch break?' When I saw the student later in the day, there was no need to ask whether he had kept the appointment. It was clear from the way he was walking!

The students had pet names for various E.E.O. personalities. Brian Youngs, because of his broad smile, was known as Monsieur Colgate, Sue Terry, caretaker and caterer, was known as Mrs. T. but the French called her Mrs. Coffee. Keith Blagrave (Peter's father) was Monsieur Puncher. The students told the story of the day he arrived in class with a heavy duty puncher. He was giving a lecture on the feet, one of his specialities, and was trying to impress upon them that feet needed air. To emphasize his point he proceeded to punch holes in their shoes! Keith was a fine osteopath, a great raconteur, and one of osteopathy's characters. Later on we had two Belgian lecturers – Jean Burnotte and Pierre Duby. The students used to enjoy showing off their knowledge of Shakespeare by saying: 'Duby… Burnotte… Duby… that is the Castejon.'

We used the conference rooms at the Royal Star Hotel in Maidstone for occasions when we needed more space such as final practical examinations. I recall setting up the room using hospital screens to create six open-ended cubicles. The exams were under way with the students (all male) wearing nothing but the briefest of briefs. Mid-morning I requested coffee for the examiners. The young cockney lass who brought it in, looked with awe at all the bronzed, scantily clad, handsome young men and exclaimed in a loud voice 'Oh... my... Gawd!' With that she dropped the tray, cups clattering and coffee splashing everywhere.

We used the Royal Star (which today is a shopping arcade) for lecturers' accommodation and many of the students stayed there as well. One evening, according to my source of information, there was an almighty soda syphon battle. It is a wonder they were not asked to leave, but then the E.E.O. was a very good customer – and soda cannot do much harm, not really.

About a year after I married Tom, I closed down my P.R. business and became instead his practice manager and generally collaborated with him in all his professional activities. It is not always easy to work with one's partner 24/7 but Tom and I did work very well together, achieving a great deal in the process, but the workload was enormous – and kept on growing. By 1972 there was no time for leisure or hobbies and even any social life was always intertwined with professional activities. Apart from the school, the I.F.P.N.T, the M.O.C., the Society of Osteopaths etc. etc. we also had *two* of everything else: two homes, two practices, two daughters, two cats – and *too* much work for *two* people!

We decided to advertise for a part-time experienced executive to share some of our workload. We were living part of the week in Sussex so Tom put an advertisement in a local newspaper on behalf of the I.F.P.N.T. as this was where help was most needed. There was a huge response but one man stood out from the rest. He had wide-ranging communication skills, plenty of high level executive experience, a great sense of humour and some part-time availability. His name was Bob Bloomfield.

The E.E.O. was flourishing but the same could not be said for the M.O.C. which had run into a number of problems with the charity commissioners. Trying to unravel all the strands was very time consuming. On the personal level, we had every sympathy for John Wernham but we felt also a great responsibility towards the students. If anything 'went wrong' we might find ourselves out on the street and without any financial backing. We sought the advice of solicitors and accountants. The advice we received was that we must cease to be a part of other organisations. Clearly the school was here to stay, and our course of action had to be to establish our own independent status.

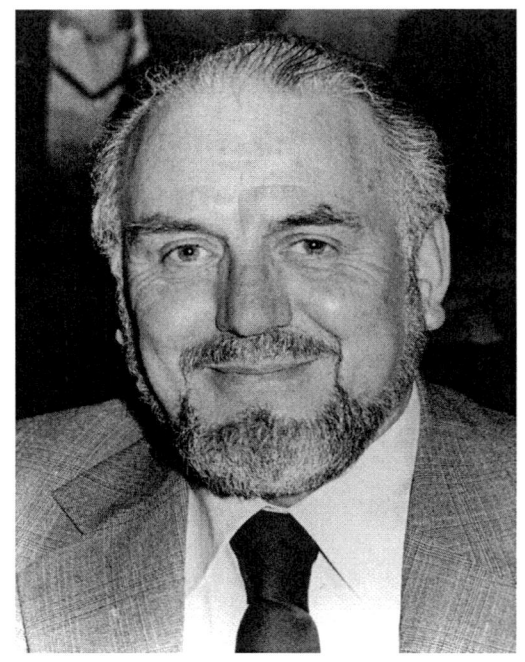

Bob Bloomfield

Things were not running smoothly for the B.N.O.A./B.C.N.O. either. There were many members of the association who felt that the college was not sufficiently accountable. Then when the newly formed Society of Osteopaths expressed the hope that there would be a close relationship with the B.N.O.A. there was a cool reception at the official level.

There was in addition considerable unrest in the B.C.N.O. among both students and faculty. The students were dissatisfied with the osteopathic element of their training. At the same time they had been well aware of the 'French School' before it relocated to Maidstone and had heard that the teaching was of a high standard.

One day when there was an E.E.O. seminar in progress, Tom and I were staying as usual in the flat at the top of 28 Tonbridge Road. Out of the blue we received a visit from Harold Klug, who was then a student at the B.C.N.O. He told us of the dissatisfaction that many of the students were feeling with their osteopathic training – and then came the big question on behalf of those students: would we consider starting a full-time osteopathic course in Maidstone?

Chapter Six

European School of Osteopathy (Maidstone)

> *'You must do the thing you think you cannot do'*
> – Eleanor Roosevelt

OSTEOPATHIC EDUCATION AND Research Ltd. was incorporated on the 19th September 1974 as a limited liability company, registered as a charity and trading as European School of Osteopathy/Ecole Européenne d'Ostéopathie – 'To promote for the public benefit the advancement of education in osteopathy.'

The unrest at the B.C.N.O. had persisted resulting in a walkout by a large group of students and a quarter of the faculty – who all headed for Maidstone. The four-year full-time diploma course started on 1st October 1974 with the former B.C.N.O. students distributed over three classes.

The students wanted to express their thanks to the Dummers for having responded to their requests. They threw a party for us at which we were presented with a beautiful wine decanter engraved with a message of gratitude to Tom and Margery. They had no idea that we were about to separate. Sadly that lovely decanter stayed in the office of the school for years, with neither of us wishing to lay claim to it. Our relationship had been on a downward slope for some 18 months. When I first knew for sure that our marriage was unravelling, the shock caused me to develop an eating disorder. My weight plummeted to six stone something and my nerves were all of a jangle.

Our professional activities – international and national – could all have been handed over if we divorced, but the school was another matter entirely. We both knew that if either of us walked away, the school would collapse – and the school was far more important than our personal problems. Advertising for a replacement was not an option because there was no money to offer. Having been a part of the B.C.N.O. and then the M.O.C., any meagre sums that had accumulated were left behind for the respective charities. Financially therefore the school was starting again from scratch, for the third time. Emotionally, I wanted to walk away from everything, but my over-developed sense of responsibility would not let me. Besides I kept remembering Cambodia.

When I was a young teenager, my father, on one of his business trips to the East, had brought me back a tablecloth. It was batik and the pattern it bore was of the temples of Angkor Wat. I did not know at the time that this was one of the most famous archaeological sites in South-East Asia and the largest religious monument in the world. It was built originally as a Hindu temple but from the 15th century it became and has remained a Buddhist shrine. All I knew was that I wanted to see it one day – and that day came when we decided that our planned trip to India would include several days in Cambodia en route from Australia. This was not long before their civil war and the tyranny of the Khmer Rouge that followed.

I have had the good fortune to see a great deal of the world, but the visit to Angkor Wat remains the most impressive and memorable experience ever. How could these extraordinary temples have been built early in the 12th century in the middle of the jungle. The sheer scale of it was astonishing. We had spent a whole day with a personal guide, marvelling at all we saw, but I wanted to go back to the temples on our own very early the next day to watch the sunrise. Tom had wandered off somewhere and I sat alone on the steps of one of the temples watching the ribbons of sunlight pierce the jungle. It was incredibly still and unbelievably peaceful. I felt at one with everything and certain that all life was related. I hope it does not sound pretentious but I can only describe it as a spiritual experience. Then out of the blue DADIRRI again – that Aboriginal quality I referred to earlier. Somewhere from that deep spring inside my being came the words 'The school is your life's work. You must never abandon it.' The words were a little bewildering at the time but they came back to me in 1974 when we had to make a decision.

Finally, we agreed to put the house on the market and separate. Divorce by mutual consent would follow in five years time. As somebody wise once said, 'You can't reheat a soufflé.' We determined nevertheless that whatever the future held we would go on working together. It was going to be difficult but I decided to grit my teeth and put Buddhist philosophy into practice; somehow we would make it work.

When I lived in Australia and during all the time I was with Tom, everybody called me Marge (or sometimes Margie) – and I hated it. In Australia all first names are shortened, as well as everyday words e.g. 'in case it turns cold bring your *cardi*', 'the cat is sleeping in his *barki*' and so forth. I saw this time of change as the ideal moment to insist that my name was Margery. Most of my family and friends got used to it – eventually.

Emotions were running high in other areas as well. Tom and John Wernham were not getting along as well as they used to. John had been pleased to have the new full-time course in Maidstone but he was disappointed when we decided that the time had come for the school to have its own separate identity and O.E. & R. Ltd. was founded. I was one of the original subscribers to the Mems. and Arts. of the new company and a friend of ours who was an accountant, Wadie Manston, was the other subscriber. The first annual general meeting was held on the 16th December 1974. I was named Company Secretary, a post I held until 2000. Wadie Manston was named Treasurer, a post he held until his death in 1997 and Tom was named President which he remained until his death in 1998.

With a brand new charity it was impossible to seek trustees by the usual means. Instead we invited friends who had benefited from treatment and who were sympathetic to what we were trying to do. The first board members were Kenneth van Barthold, concert pianist and musicologist, David Daly theatrical agent, and Jean-Claude Faure French businessman living in England. When I think back, they were a wonderfully supportive and encouraging board.

Running seminars for the E.E.O. was one thing but now running a full-time school with all its ramifications was another thing altogether. For myself, it felt as if everything I had done previously in my P.R. career had been a great preparation for running the E.S.O. The basic principles of managing a successful business, whether it is I.C.I. or a one-man band remain the same, so running my own P.R. business was all useful experience on which I could draw. I had developed a useful talent for budgeting and financial control, both essential for the future development of the school. Tom, by his own admission, was hopeless at finance and not too keen on administration either.

Given our personal circumstances, it was helpful that we had clearly defined roles. Tom was an outstandingly gifted practitioner and he was the osteopathic inspiration for the school and in charge of curriculum development. My role was finance, administration and promotion. Between us we had enough skills until experience taught us the rest. It was a steep learning curve.

It was time now for me to give up my other activities in order to be present full-time in the school. In spite of the lack of money and all the other teething problems, there was a great atmosphere, a feeling of all being in it together, a real pioneering spirit. Expectations so far as facilities were concerned were not high. Surviving was what mattered.

Students' lack of money in those early days resulted in some unusual accommodation solutions. One I recall slept in a haystack on his first night in Kent, another in a tent, two in a caravan and yet another in my office. I would not have known about the latter but for finding his cast-off knickers and socks under my desk! After a week or two they all found themselves somewhere to live and settled down to their studies. Quite a few had to take menial part-time jobs in order to make ends meet. Not ideal, but if needs must. A number of the students were unable to transfer their grants and so it was necessary to put certain fees on the slate. As a matter of interest, the fees for our first academic year were £175! Faculty members were uncomplaining when I often had to ask them to wait for payment of their modest lecturing fees. In fact *everyone* was so understanding of the financial pressures and struggles to get the full-time course established.

Because, initially, we were so small, there was great communication with the students. We listened to their ideas and if they were good and affordable, we introduced them. One such was the Christmas Revue which continues to this day. It gives the students, and some faculty as well, the opportunity 'to take the mickey'. There are many images that will live forever in my memory. I recall sitting next to John and Jess Wernham when Clive Lindley-Jones did an impersonation of J.W. I had never seen them laugh so much. Clive was more like John than John. Then there was David Melrose in an apron, pretending to be Sue Terry, with a black fur around his neck representing Sam her black cat. Mark Young made a well observed Tom and Mervyn Waldman was memorable for his virtually horizontal exit from the stage, earning him the title of 'Super-Merv'. At a later Revue Simon Fielding in fishnets and Tony Norrie in, well, nothing except a spinal column were equally memorable.

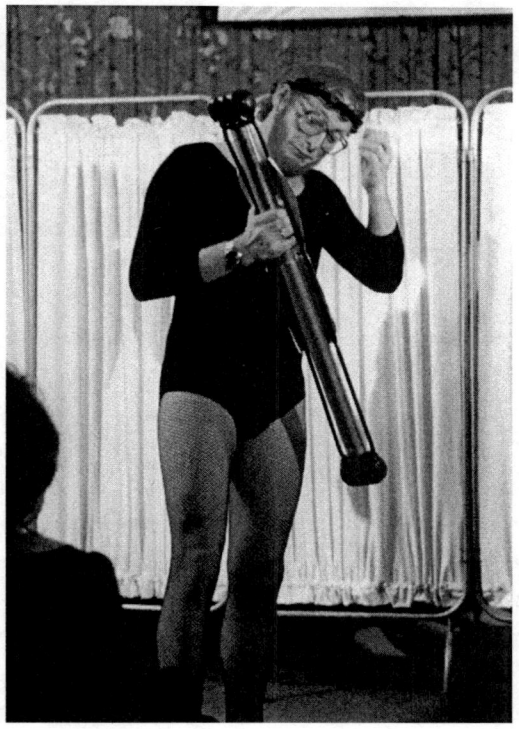

Simon Fielding – in fishnets

In setting up the company we emphasized in the Memorandum the international aspirations of the school. We envisaged it as an international centre of osteopathic excellence – and that was how it developed. When my telephone rang it could be a prospective student from anywhere in the world – South

America, Hawaii, Australia, Singapore – anywhere and everywhere. We never advertised – so how did people hear about us? It was all word of mouth. Graduates of the E.E.O./E.S.O. would sing the praises of the school on trips abroad or through personal contacts in various countries.

Among my personal archives I have come across a letter from the accountant in which

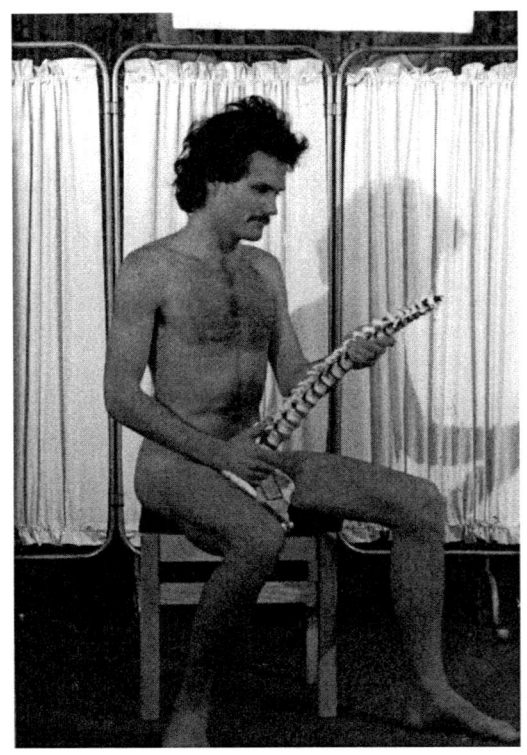

Tony Norrie – in a spinal column

he refers to my first 'employment' by O.E. & R. Ltd. on 17th September 1978. I remember how chuffed I was to receive my first very own pay packet – not so much for the money as for the clear indication that the school was able at last to afford to pay me something however small. From the outset Tom had drawn a very modest principal's fee which, in theory, was supposed to cover my services as well. Rather reminiscent of that quotable quote from some computer buff – 'In theory there is no difference between theory and practice. But in practice there is.' The thing about starting a charity without any funding is that you *know* it is going to be tough going – but if you believe in it totally, you *know* also that it is worth it – and eventually all will be well.

By 1978 we had over 20 different nationalities in the school. Together with the part-time course, there were now over 300 students enrolled and space was again a problem. We were having overflow seminars in the Royal Star Hotel. John Wernham looked into the possibility of building in the garden at the back of No. 28 Tonbridge Road. Tom explored the feasibility of a London clinic. I set about looking for property in the vicinity (and pondering how on earth we would pay for it). I seem to recall it was Martin Booth who spotted that 104 Tonbridge Road was up for sale. We viewed the property, and decided there and then it would be ideal.

As our sponsoring company, O.E. & R. Ltd. was not very old, it proved to be impossible to persuade anyone to give us a 100% mortgage. I was getting desperate. I remember Robert (Bloomfield – we were now living together) saying to me 'When you come to the end of the rope, darling, tie a knot and hang on.' I did just that. The following week J.W. popped into my office and said 'I see no reason why my charity can't give your charity a loan to buy that property. Come upstairs and we'll sort it out.' What a relief. I could hardly believe it.

I was able to get the price reduced by £10,000 – and we signed on the dotted line. 104 Tonbridge Road had belonged to the Kent and Sussex Farmers' Union. The building had been empty for nearly two years. There was a huge amount of work to be done, much of it before we could even think about moving in. Roof repairs, complete re-wiring, central heating installation, plumbing, as well as meeting all the building and fire regulations. Tremendous expenditure was on the horizon so there had to be even stricter financial control plus fundraising – and unshakeable faith in the future!

Looking through my fundraising archives I have just come across a leaflet for a fundraising piano recital by our friend and board member Kenneth van Barthold. It was held on 27th January 1979 in the beautiful banqueting hall of Allington Castle, followed by a champagne supper. As luck would have it, there was a heavy fall of snow that afternoon and evening which reduced the anticipated audience, but for those who managed to get there it was a magical evening of Chopin.

Before moving into 104 Tonbridge Road, there were a number of break-ins. The building works in progress included complete re-wiring. The electrician was angered by the fact that he would do a day's work only to come in the next morning and find all the wiring had been ripped out. On the fourth break-in, I received a telephone call from the police about 1am (I was always a key holder for the school) saying they had caught a tramp on the premises. Apparently he had lifted a couple of floorboards in the main hall, stuffed newspapers underneath and then set fire to the paper. Fortunately the police had arrived on the scene before it was a serious blaze. It turned out to be the same man who had broken in each time as he was trying desperately to get caught! He wanted to spend the winter in gaol because he found it too cold living on the streets. How very sad.

At long last the school had its own premises – a defining moment – but there was still a lot of work to be done and so little money with which to do it. J.W. waived the interest on our mortgage for the first year which was much appreciated but I still had a long shopping list – carpets, curtains, treatment tables, chairs, desks etc. – and there was still the whole building to be redecorated inside. We decided to cancel lectures for a week but students and faculty were asked to come in as usual. The idea was to give the place a thorough cleaning and redecorate as much as possible.

Robert undertook the task of getting it all organised – and he did it with military precision. The 'task force' was individually

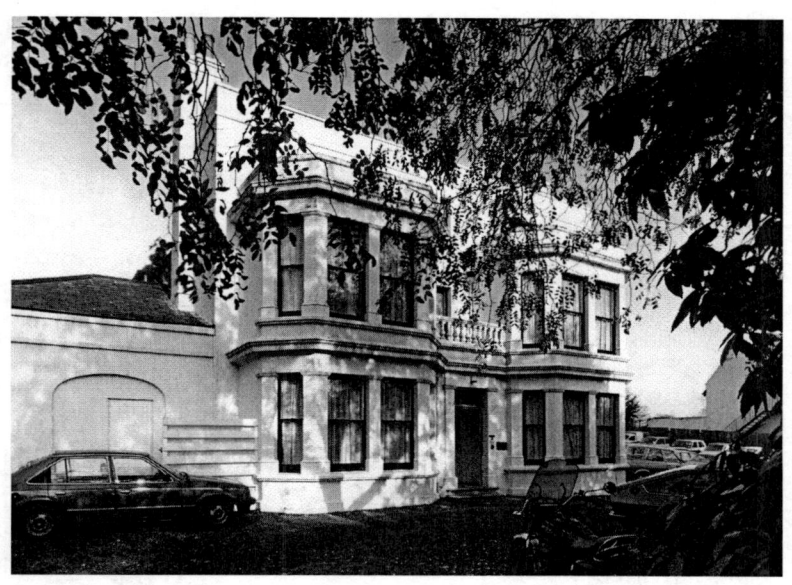

104 Tonbridge Road

assessed so that the jobs to be done could be matched to ability (where it existed!). Even sandwich and tea making were appropriately allocated. It was such a fun week – but we did achieve a lot as well. I have vivid memories of, for example, Stephen Pirie wielding a paint brush clad in torn, cast-off trousers held together with very large safety pins; John Stevens balancing precariously on top of a tall ladder in the stairwell; Johnny Mickerson frighteningly in charge of a blow torch. Clive Lindley-Jones, Elizabeth Davenport-Fry and Margery swept out the large and filthy cellar – coal, unwanted Farmers' Union files and dead mice. Then there was Khaled Ben Moussa who painted the toilets in a sort of pee yellow, and Piers Chandler covered passageway walls in a high gloss white paint. Yes, we did make a few mistakes but not nearly as many as when I allowed a student free reign on colour schemes. He claimed to have been an interior designer before becoming an E.S.O. student and, stupidly, I believed him. So there were a few jobs that had to be done again but, overall, we saved a lot of money and in the end there was a feeling of 'Well, we have put our mark on the building.'

When the time came to move in, April 1979, we decided to save money by doing the removal ourselves and hired a van. Robert, myself and two students (one of whom was Simon Fielding) carried out the task.

Once we were settled in, my aim was to create a cheerful, welcoming ambience. There were always fresh flowers in the en-

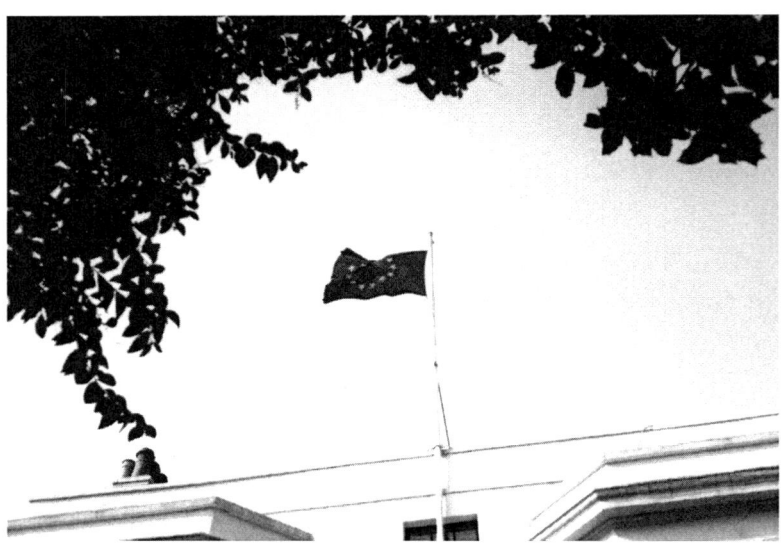

The School's own flag – the logo inside Europe

trance hall, warm colours, and pictures on the wall. In addition I had alternative concealed lighting installed in the main hall so that the atmosphere could be transformed for evening events. Small details perhaps but I believed that a pleasant ambience was conducive to the learning process.

The official opening of 104 Tonbridge Road was performed by Dr John Upledger. It took place on 7th July 1979 and was coupled with a Society of Osteopaths Conference. The Belgian osteopathic society presented us with the School's own European flag – and fortunately we had a flag pole on top of the building from which to fly it.

A medal of honour was presented to Paul Gény, without whom the school in Paris would not have existed. A medal of honour was presented also to John Wernham in recognition of all the help and support he had given the school.

On the personal level things were still a bit difficult, but improving. Life has a habit of moving on. Tom was now living with Jo Bradbury (Parnell's widow) and I was living with Robert Bloomfield as previously mentioned. Sometimes there were even comical moments. One such was when we all had to attend a conference in Brussels. The Belgian osteopathic society sent flowers to the hotel where they had booked our accommodation. When the bouquets arrived, the hall porter was totally confused. To which rooms should they be delivered? Why was Mrs Dummer sharing a room with Mr Bloomfield, while Mr Dummer was sharing a room with Mrs Bradbury? A good question!

In 1979 Tom married Jo, and I married Robert. Doesn't life play funny tricks!

Chapter Seven

Society of Osteopaths
The Genesis Osteopathic Foundation

'The whole is only as good as the sum total of its parts'

THE OSTEOPATHIC PROFESSION was in disarray. The G.C. and R.O. had *not* succeeded in registering all competent osteopaths, in fact by the 1970s there were probably more competent osteopaths outside the G.C. and R.O. than there were on it.

In order to try and break the deadlock, a group of osteopaths decided to found a new organisation in the hope that it would act as a unifying influence. On the 22nd December 1971 the Society of Osteopaths (limited by guarantee) was incorporated.

The following information is taken from various Society publications:

It had a small founder membership consisting of members, ex-members or graduates of the B.C.N.O./B.N.O.A. and a smaller number of graduates of the B.S.O. The Society also had roots in its association with the Maidstone Osteopathic Clinic and the former Osteopathic Institute of Applied Technique both of which sought to preserve important aspects of our osteopathic heritage. The Society was therefore a somewhat eclectic organisation. Initially, it sought to fulfil two important needs. The first was to establish a non-political learned body dedicated to the preservation of the identity of osteopathy, in its purest and most complete form. The second need – consistent with the first – was to form a grouping that would dissociate itself from any suggestion that osteopathy was a musculo-skeletal adjunct to either conventional medicine or naturopathy.

With the emergence of the E.S.O. and its teaching in 1974, the Society soon acquired its direction and identity, concerning itself with a broadly based and highly osteopathic orientation which was reflected in its meetings and conferences. The D.O. of the E.S.O. became the standard for full members.

During the next decade it attracted many distinguished speakers and fostered conferences of a high standard. Early

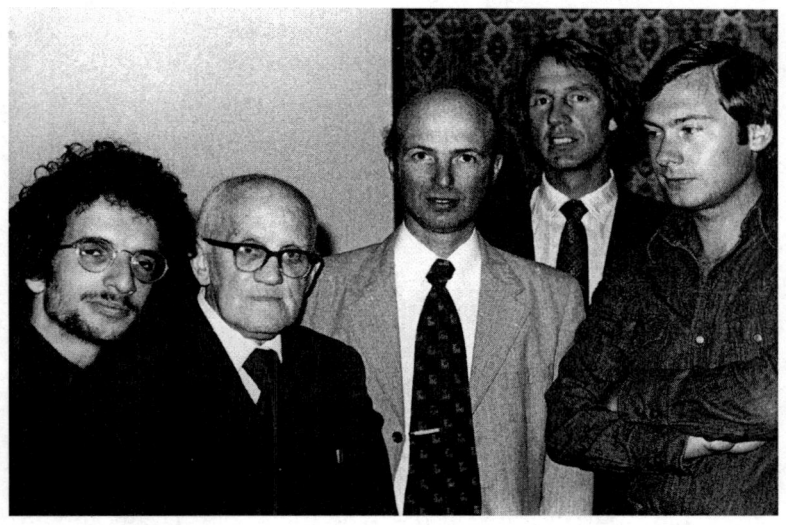

L – R: Alain Abehsera, Willis Haycock, Harold Klug, Ron Cook and Robert Lever

on it centred more on the classical exponents – T.E. Hall and John Wernham. Willis Haycock introduced functional technique, Denis Brookes brought the cranial orientation, which was further expounded by John Upledger, Professor at Michigan State University College of Osteopathic Medicine, who became a frequent visitor. I shall never forget calling in at the Society of Osteopaths meeting which was being held at Hendon Hall in North London on the first occasion Dr John Upledger lectured. The atmosphere in the room was unlike any other gathering of osteopaths that I had experienced. Everyone looked 'spaced out' and yet at the same time full of wonderment, as if they had just been given the most amazing gift. I guess that was exactly what was happening. John Upledger subsequently established an undergraduate programme for the E.S.O. introducing senior students to the cranio-sacral approach.

The Society was also active in building relationships with the profession in the U.S.A. In September 1981 the first Anglo-American conference was organised by the Society of Osteopaths in co-operation with the E.S.O. and the Michigan Center for Continuing Education in Osteopathic Medicine. This was a highly successful event and paved the way for many more American colleagues who came to lecture at the E.S.O. and/or Society conferences.

The Society published an excellent journal ably edited by Harold Klug and Robert Lever. It came out twice a year – spring and autumn – and copies were given to all E.S.O. students.

The ever increasing political issues besetting the profession were of great concern to the Society. If osteopathy was to grow and flourish then professional unity was paramount. The Society and the E.S.O. determined to build bridges especially with the B.S.O. and the G.C. and R.O. Over the second half of the '70s many meetings were held although probably the most progress was made through personal contacts. Getting to know each other's standards was an important step in bringing the profession together and to this end reciprocal visits between the E.S.O. and the B.S.O. were arranged.

These closer relations finally led to a meeting, on 25th February 1980, when Tom and I met with the principal and academic head of the B.S.O. There was unanimous agreement that in the interests of unity for the profession, the major osteopathic bodies had to get together. A decision was taken that the E.S.O. would seek accreditation of its four-year full-time course by the G.C. and R.O. The B.S.O. offered help and support. It was hugely satisfying to witness barriers crumbling and prejudices fading away. In 1982 there was a successful outcome to the G.C. and R.O.'s inspection of the E.S.O. which was announced officially in 1983.

Up until this point the school's registering body had been the Society of Osteopaths. Now it was time for the Society to transfer its regulatory function to the G.C. and R.O. as all E.S.O. graduates were eligible for membership of the Register along with all other Society members. At the same time it was agreed that representatives of the Society would sit on the executive council of the G.C. and R.O. Professional unity and co-operation had taken a very big step forward.

The Society of Osteopaths now reverted to its academic role as a postgraduate body as well as the school's alumni, and thus it remained until the early 1990s when it was decided that the Society had fulfilled all its objectives and was no longer necessary. By this time the E.S.O. had an active and highly successful postgraduate department. Agreement was reached that the school was to take over the Society as its alumni organisation.

There is no doubt that the Society of Osteopaths together with the E.S.O. played a pivotal role in the development of osteopathy in the U.K. Another body about which the same could be said is The Genesis Osteopathic Foundation although its function was totally different.

Genesis was registered as a charity in 1980 to promote research into osteopathy and to assist osteopathic education, and in particular the E.S.O. The original trustees were Harold Klug, Robert Lever and Jack Taylor who were all on the executive committee of the society and lecturers at the E.S.O. Later Simon Fielding became a trustee. There were also honorary patrons of the trust: Tom Dummer, who at the time was president of the Society as well as principal of the school, Professor John Upledger of the Michigan State University College of Osteopathic Medicine and Dr Dudley Tee, Head of the

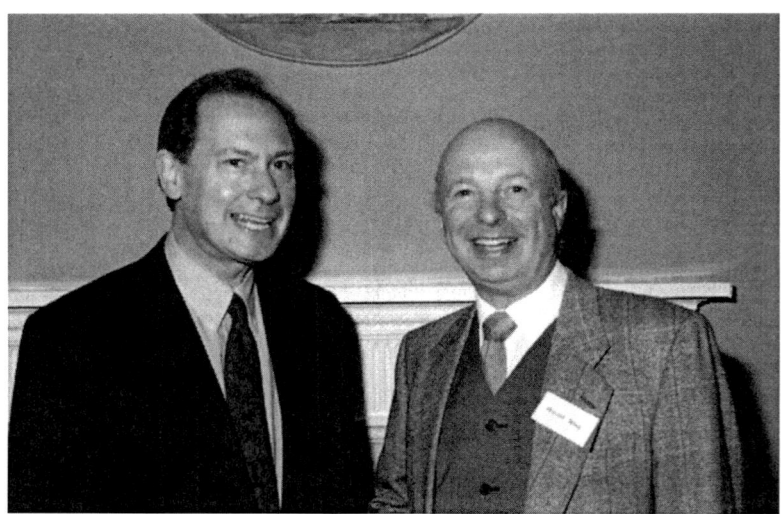

L – R: Robert Lever and Harold Klug

Department of Immunology and Vice Dean of Kings College Hospital Medical School, London.

Looking through my file of correspondence with Genesis, I feel so grateful for all the help and support they gave the school over the years. Harold Klug, Robert Lever and Simon Fielding were always very discreet about the work of Genesis but I know it helped fund all the expenses that were involved in the whole process of going for statutory regulation. They worked tirelessly for the profession in so many different areas.

Chapter Eight

Politics and Politicians

> 'Politics is the gentle art of getting votes from the poor and campaign funds from the rich by promising to protect each from the other'
> – Oscar Ameringer

ONE DAY IN the late 1960s we received a telephone call from the Right Honourable Ernest Marples M.P. (Minister of Transport). He had heard about the school and our connections with France and invited us to his home to discuss an idea he had. This was the beginning of a friendship with Ernest and his wife Ruth, and the start of a very interesting project.

They had a house in Fleuri, France, right in the middle of vineyards and nearby they had also bought a magnificent château called Château de Chaintré. He wanted to explore the possibility of turning it into a health home specialising in osteopathic treatment.

Ernest invited us to Fleuri to stay with them for a few days during which we could view the château and see what we thought of its potential as a health home. Working with Ernest was a fascinating experience.

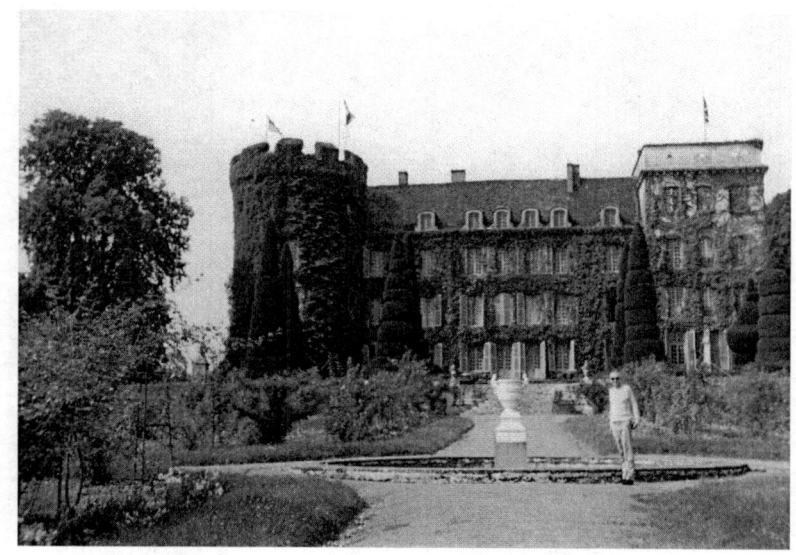

Château de Chaintré

The next step was to set up a meeting and we enlisted the help of Ange Castejon in Lyon who made contact with all the local osteopaths. The plan was to meet at the château, give our views and discuss the possibilities with Ernest.

Needless to say some wine tasting followed the meeting, with samples from the château's vast wine cellars.

Sketches were prepared of the alterations that would be necessary and a plan of action gradually evolved. There were many meetings plus further trips to France.

The big problem, however, was the illegal situation of osteopathy. Even with all the influence Ernest had, it proved to be impossible to obtain the necessary permissions and unfortunately the project had to be abandoned.

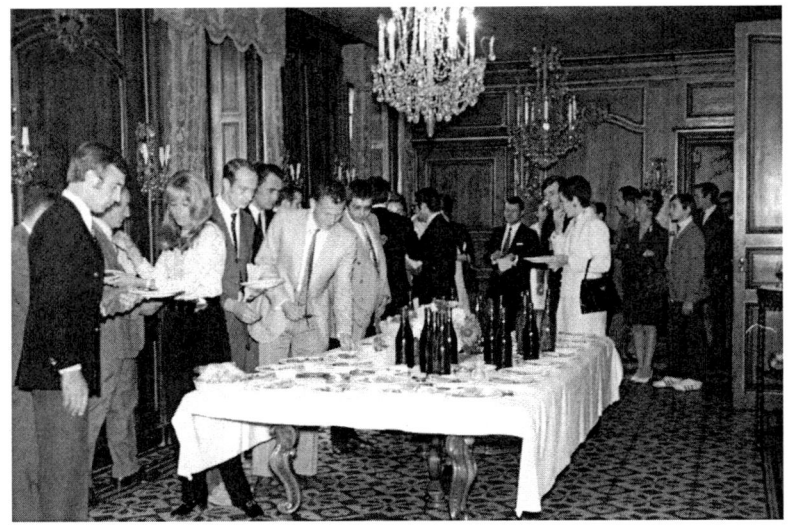

A gathering of French osteopaths at the Château for discussions with Ernest Marples

Over the years Ernest Marples proved to be a good friend of the natural therapeutics movement, always willing to offer help, advice and support. He was personally health conscious too; for example, I recall that sometimes he would jog over from his home in SW1 to our practice near Baker Street where he would arrive in good time for his treatment from Tom. I remember also a splendid dinner that he hosted at the House of Commons for practitioners and their partners.

Mrs Joyce Butler, M.P. was another staunch supporter. In my personal archives I have found my invitation to another House of Commons dinner which she sponsored for the B.N.O.A. to celebrate the 21st anniversary of their college. This was held on 10th October 1970.

Due to the good offices of both Ernest Marples and Joyce Butler, in 1973 some meetings were held at the House of Commons to explore the possibility of setting up a political

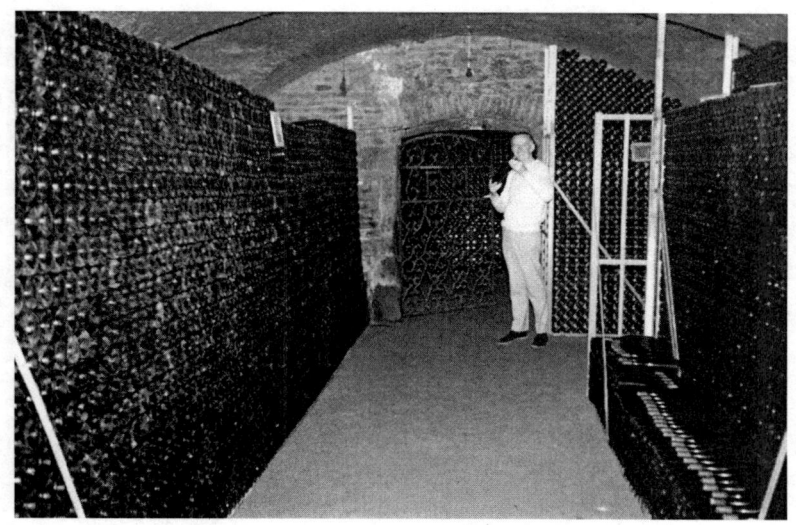

Just a corner of the cellars at the Château

defence committee which could coordinate a lobby in case of legislation arising from the E.E.C. Nine British natural therapeutic organisations participated – including the Osteopathic Association of Great Britain (O.A.G.B.) although, after the second meeting, they withdrew preferring to 'go it alone' rather than associate with this particular group.

Later in the 1970s there was much debate about whether the profession should go for registration of osteopathy under the Professions Supplementary to Medicine Act 1960. Finally it was considered to be a 'bad idea'. I have in my files interesting correspondence that passed between Dr David Owen (then Minister of Health), Mrs Joyce Butler and my husband Robert, at that point in his capacity as secretary of the Paramedical Practitioners Committee for Natural Therapeutics (P.P.C.N.T.)

Another M.P. was becoming involved again, Tony Durant, who had been of immense help with The International Federation

(I.F.P.N.T.). Tony was an old friend of Robert's who, as I shall reveal later, played a pivotal role in the regulation of osteopathy.

In 1976, with much encouragement from the B.N.O.A., Mrs Joyce Butler M.P. (Wood Green) introduced a Bill to provide for the registration of osteopaths, but it failed at the second reading on objection. Apparently senior civil servants had found out that the osteopathic profession was fragmented and that only one section had encouraged Mrs Butler with her Bill. As far as the other groups were concerned, the feeling was that the Bill was premature. Unity had to be achieved before seeking any form of statutory regulation (rather reminiscent of everything the International Federation had pushed for over many years!).

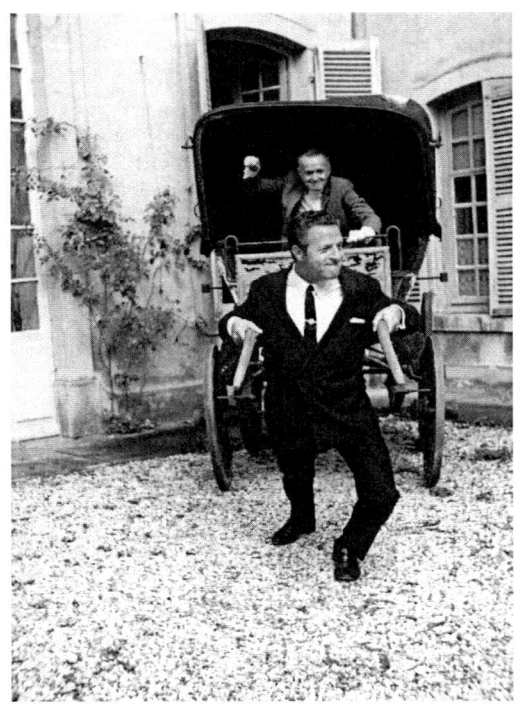

In the Château courtyard – Tom in the carriage with Ange Castejon 'horsing about'

Perhaps it is time to introduce a little light relief before continuing the story of osteopathic legislation in this country. During my travels with Tom we met up with a number of M.P.s in various countries, always taking the opportunity to introduce the work of the I.F.P.N.T.

In Australia we met the Honourable Mr Douglas Darby, Member of the Legislative Assembly in New South Wales. We were taken to lunch at a fish restaurant followed by a preview of Sydney Opera House, which had not yet been opened officially. We arrived just as they were completing the carpet laying in the vast front foyer. It was an amazing colour – rich dark purple and very thick. As we walked across the carpet, I suddenly felt very sick. I recall it was a blazing hot day and it was obvious that I had eaten something at lunch which was heralding the onset of food poisoning. I made a wild dash for the loo on the far side of the foyer – but didn't make it! What a way to christen that beautiful carpet. I have never felt so embarrassed.

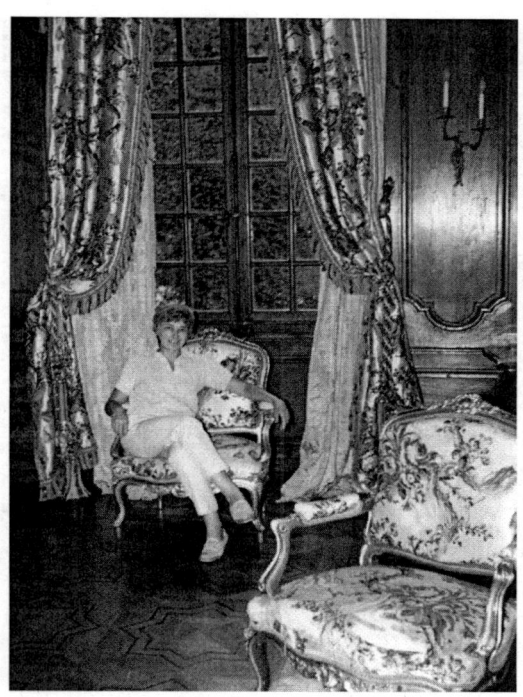

Margery relaxing in the Salon at the Château

Now let us turn back the clock. Osteopathy first came to Great Britain in 1898 by way of some lectures delivered by Dr J. Martin Littlejohn, star pupil of the Founder of Osteopathy, Dr A.T. Still. Later a number of graduates of American colleges settled over here, and by 1911 there was a sufficient number of

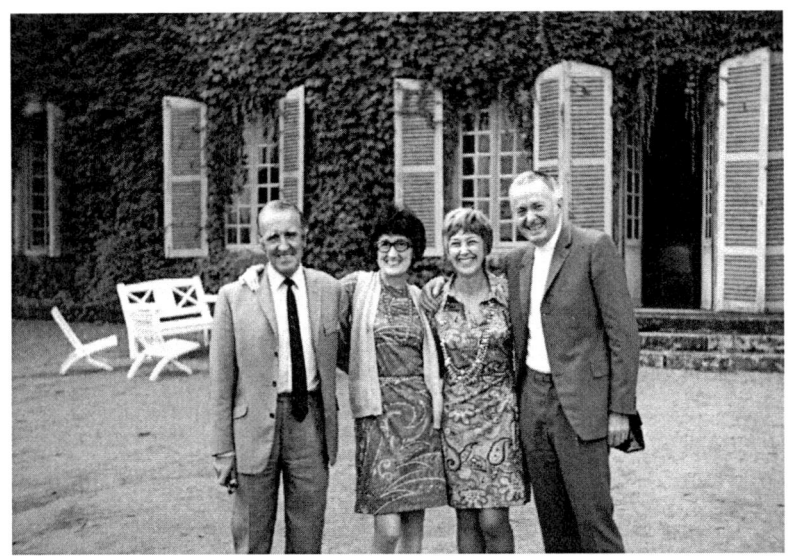

L – R: Ernest and Ruth Marples, Margery and Tom on the terrace of the Château

them to form the first osteopathic association in this country – the British Osteopathic Association. J. Martin Littlejohn (J.M.L.) returned to settle permanently in this country in 1913 and, in 1917, he founded the British School of Osteopathy.

I do not propose to go into *all* the attempts to achieve statutory regulation for osteopathy, but the following endeavour is of particular significance. In 1931 a Bill to regulate osteopathy was introduced into the House of Commons by a Mr W.M. Adamson (Kennock). It failed but a few years later Robert Boothby introduced it as a Private Members' Bill. Late in 1934 Viscount Elibank took it to the House of Lords and from there it was referred to a Select Committee. It was found in 1935, that there was not a sufficiently strong case at that time to adopt the Bill's proposals.

In a memorandum from the Ministry of Health dated 8th

April 1935, it was suggested that if osteopaths were unhappy with their status they could either train to become doctors and join the medical register, or set up a voluntary register of osteopaths along with effective training institutions.

The latter course of action was preferred and on 22nd July 1936 a voluntary register was incorporated under the title of the General Council and Register of Osteopaths. It is interesting to conjecture that if the G.C. and R.O. had not been so intransigent in its attitude to osteopaths outside its jurisdiction then perhaps unity *and* statutory recognition would have come sooner; however, playing the 'if' game is pointless. The fact is that the profession had to wait until 1993 for the Osteopaths Act.

During the late 1970s my husband Robert had a number of articles published on osteopathy in which he urged the profession to start thinking seriously about the kind of legislation that would suit them – and then pursue it before a 'legislative solution' got thrust upon them from elsewhere, an elsewhere indeed that might be hostile to their very existence. We were discussing these thoughts over dinner one evening when Robert posed the question 'Who, out of all the osteopaths we know, would be the one most likely to be interested in – and ultimately successful – in pursuing legislation for osteopathy?' We lapsed into pensive mode for a while and then both of us came up with the same name: Simon Fielding. Simon was still a student at the time (1979) in his fourth and final year at the E.S.O. 'Yes,' he told Robert, he 'would be interested.' The plan was that when he graduated he would get himself on to the council of the G.C. and R.O. and then at some suitable moment he would raise the question of legislation. I understand that he did so on several occasions without result. Finally, perhaps tiring of the question coming up yet again, the chairman asked Simon to go away and research the various possible courses of action and then report back. In the meantime Robert had been in touch with his friend since Royal Navy days, Tony Durant M.P. It was agreed that Robert would take Simon to meet Tony over lunch at the House of Commons – and this was how it all started.

It was a long and tortuous road between that meeting in the House and the achievement of the Osteopaths Act 1993 – 'to regulate the education, training and practice of osteopaths.' Throughout those long years Tony Durant (later to become Sir Anthony Durant) gave freely of his advice, help and support and, finally, was one of the sponsors of the Bill.

It is not for me to write of all the ups and downs of the long journey to the Osteopaths Act 1993 but it is my hope that one day Simon Fielding will find the time to record the fascinating story for posterity.

Chapter Nine

European School of Osteopathy

> *'Education is not the filling of a bucket,*
> *but the lighting of a fire'*
> – W.B. Yeats

THE MOMENT WE moved into our new premises at 104 Tonbridge Road, vast though they seemed by comparison, I realised that they were not going to be big enough in a couple of years time. I persuaded an architect friend to walk around the property with me and discuss the various ideas I had for expansion. Everything was possible providing we could pay for it. Planning ahead was essential – at least three years at a time was the policy. In the 1980s we gradually developed the site, building a clinic, an extension to the main lecture hall, additional classroom in the garden, enlarged kitchen, canteen and laundry facilities, and a first floor extension for offices.

The osteopathic teaching at the E.S.O. reflected a broad spectrum of the subject. Tom was determined that the academic climate would be liberal. Although students were expected to accept the fundamental principles and apply their studies accordingly, nevertheless they were encouraged to think originally and express their ideas in an atmosphere of academic freedom. The patient was the unifying theme of the educational programme – and the sole reason for our existence.

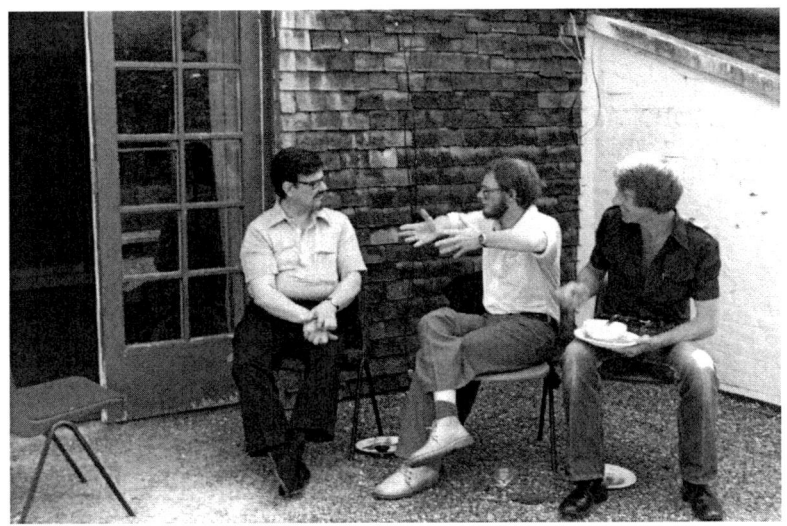

L – R: Fred Mitchell Jr., Simon Fielding, Ron Cook

Dr John Upledger was now a regular lecturer at the school and many other American colleagues followed. Fred Mitchell Jr. had a three-week stay with us during which he introduced Mitchell Technique to both faculty and students. Larry Jones followed introducing counterstrain technique. Greatly appreciated too were Viola Frymann's lectures.

Visits from Dr Irvin (Kim) Korr, distinguished physiologist and health promotion crusader were always memorable. Kim was a professor at Texas College of Osteopathic Medicine. Prior to that he had spent some 30 years at Kirksville where he had encountered osteopathic philosophy for the first time which, he claimed, had changed the course of his life. His lectures were always full of warmth, wisdom and humour, like the man himself.

Members of the French faculty lectured on the full-time course as well, such as Jean-Pierre Barral with his important

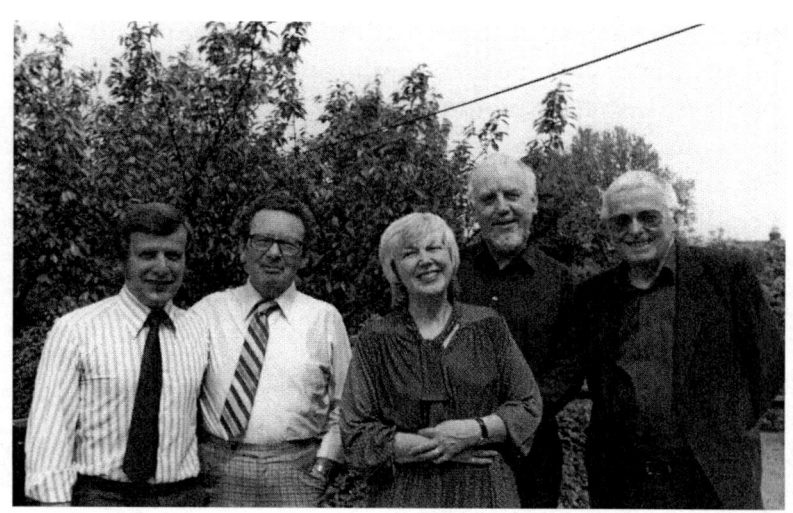

L – R: John Barkworth, Kim Korr,
Robert and Margery and Tom

contribution in visceral technique which was yet another highlight. There was always an air of excitement when we welcomed guest lecturers – and there were many of them. The E.S.O. embraced American and European influences. The input both from the U.S.A. and from our colleagues across the Channel brought a richness to the teaching, which could not be bettered.

We organised some staff exchanges with American universities in the late 1980s and '90s which were appreciated by all concerned – and then there was that memorable visitor introduced to us by John Upledger. Her name was Sister Anne Brooks, an osteopathic medical student at Michigan State University who spent two months in Europe on an elective in osteopathy. The religious order to which she belonged allowed the sisters to go out into the world and qualify in an area of their choice provided their newly acquired skill could be used in the future to help people.

Sister Anne attended lectures at the E.S.O. for several weeks followed by some time spent in the practices of various D.O.s. Neither the students nor the lecturers were at all fazed by having a nun in the class. She wore jeans and sweaters and looked like any other student, with a sense of fun to match. We hosted her attendance at an International Osteopathic Congress in Brussels, and then Robert and I drove her to La Poizat in France where John Upledger was giving a cranial course and she was able to act as a table assistant for him.

When Sister Anne qualified from Michigan State University, she looked for the poorest, most deprived town in the U.S.A. and there she set up her osteopathic clinic. I understand she is doing some wonderful work.

I have often remarked that during the four years of osteopathic training, students change quite a lot – and of course, for the better! During the early days of the school, some of the students displayed outward signs of change as well, almost as if they were trying to find their true identity. All shall be nameless. For example there were those who changed their names – and not just by marriage. One student changed names three times in four years (come to think of it even I went from Marge to Margery!).

Then there were those male students who either grew a beard – or shaved one off, grew their hair long – or shaved it off and some of course just went bald! I found it fascinating to observe the changes – on *all* levels. I suppose it could be said that during the four years of osteopathic studies, some students simply 'grew up' – whatever age they were when they started – and we did tend to attract far more mature applicants in the early days, most of whom had decided on a change of career following a personal experience of the benefits of osteopathic treatment.

There were many E.S.O. romances, a considerable number of which led to marriage. I lost count of how many weddings I attended. Some osteopathic marriages lasted – and some did not… but that's life.

Something that has been happening for quite a long time now, is that we have second generation graduates, which is great.

For me there were two highlights in each academic year – the first and last days. Induction Day was so special, seeing all the new students and reflecting on the journey they were about to start. We gave them loads of information and advice, and reminded them of much that had been said during their initial interviews. For example, it was 'hands on' from day one which meant stripping down to the underwear. I understand Marks and Spencer did a roaring trade in knickers during the late afternoon of Induction Day. In the evening we held a party to welcome the new first years to which all the other students were invited as well. It was a great social gathering to kick-start the new academic session.

Graduation Day was a day of celebration, tinged with a little sadness that we were saying 'au revoir' to so many students. In the early days our graduation ceremonies were rather informal – with loads of hugging when the diplomas were presented – but students and their families and friends loved them. We would start off with the graduating year and staff having champagne and smoked salmon on the terrace outside my office. Then we would be joined downstairs by everyone else for the presentation of diplomas, and speeches. This was followed by strawberries and cream provided by the graduating students, and wine provided by the school. Later we introduced an evening event as well which over time became a graduation ball organised by the students. When we moved on to degree status the graduation

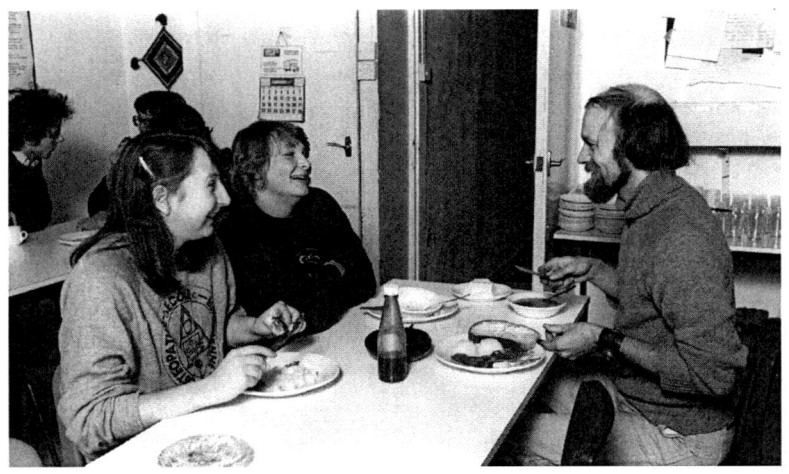

Guess who the man on the right is...

ceremony became more formal of course but it remains such a happy day. I have never missed one.

Having the clinical training at the Maidstone Osteopathic Clinic, just a few minutes away, worked quite well to start with, but gradually the relationship began to unravel. The hostility between Tom and J.W. grew. I was always trying to keep the peace and smooth the considerably ruffled feathers. J.W. disapproved of Tom's specific adjusting technique referring to it as 'chiropractic', hotly denied by Tom of course. J.W. would not allow it to be practised in his clinic, in fact he would not allow anything other than his own approach, and this was the crux of the problem.

The school's osteopathic canvas was broad although J.W.'s approach constituted a major part of the teaching. It soon became a source of frustration to the students who could not practise clinically the full range of everything they were being taught in the classroom. Some of them were getting a bit rebellious and would turn up late for their clinic sessions. Understandably, this would infuriate J.W. who would then shout down the 'phone at me about the students' lack of discipline, even suggesting that the school should have a change of principal. On a really bad day J.W. would threaten to call in the mortgage.

In spite of all, I had a good personal relationship with John, as did Robert, and we met with him many times, just as friends, to try and sort out the problems. I could appreciate fully that he wanted *his* clinic run *his* way, of course he did, but understanding his point of view did nothing to help resolve matters. In addition we were concerned about the clinic's facilities. John was not one to spend his charity's money 'needlessly'. As a result things had become very shabby and not of the standard that we felt was appropriate for a fast growing osteopathic school. Size was also a consideration; more treatment rooms would be needed in the near future.

Tom, by this time, had withdrawn from all discussions of the problem. He asked Stephen Pirie to take up correspondence with J.W. Peter Blagrave also tried, but we were not getting anywhere, so it was decided to invite J.W. to a meeting in a final attempt to resolve our difficulties. John refused to attend – and there were more threats to call in the mortgage. Clearly things were reaching an all time low. Then we heard that J.W. had offered a substantial sum of money to the B.S.O. appeal, in full knowledge of how hard the E.S.O. still had to struggle financially. The B.S.O. did not accept the offer. A parting of the ways was inevitable and on the 2nd June 1981 we wrote severing our relationship with the M.O.C. It fell to me to write the letter and I must say I did so with a heavy heart. In order to avoid disruption for patients we said that our students and tutors would continue to man the clinic until such time as John could make alternative arrangements. In the autumn of 1981 John Wernham opened the Maidstone College of Osteopathy.

Osteopathic schools and clinics are few and far between in the U.K., yet in Maidstone, Kent we were about to have two of each within a few minutes of each other. How crazy – and how sad that our two charities, with so much in common, did not succeed in working together. Years later I tried again but more of that in Chapter 11.

Fortunately, by 1981, the school had an impressive record of growth and achievement, and it was not difficult to transfer the loan from the M.O.C. to Barclays Bank. Our next problem however was to provide – as soon as possible – the clinical training for our students.

We started an embryo clinic in the school building, during the evenings, when the space was available. As another interim solution, the B.S.O. offered facilities for the E.S.O. to have a unit of students and tutors within the B.S.O.'s London clinic, which was due to start in May. Unbelievably, the G.C. and R.O. objected to the proposed arrangement and it had to be postponed. After further discussions between the B.S.O. and the Register agreement was reached, and the E.S.O. unit began in autumn 1981. This cooperation between the two schools plus an exchange of lecturers and then co-examining all contributed to a greater understanding between the B.S.O. and the E.S.O.

During the summer holiday period of 1981, whilst the space was available in the school, Tom and Stephen Pirie worked tirelessly to build up a base of clinic patients. When the new academic year began, we had sorted out ways of juggling our space to allow for the clinic activity to continue – but every room had to double up its use, which was far from ideal.

The next challenge for the E.S.O. was to have its own clinic. I had been hunting for local properties ever since our split with

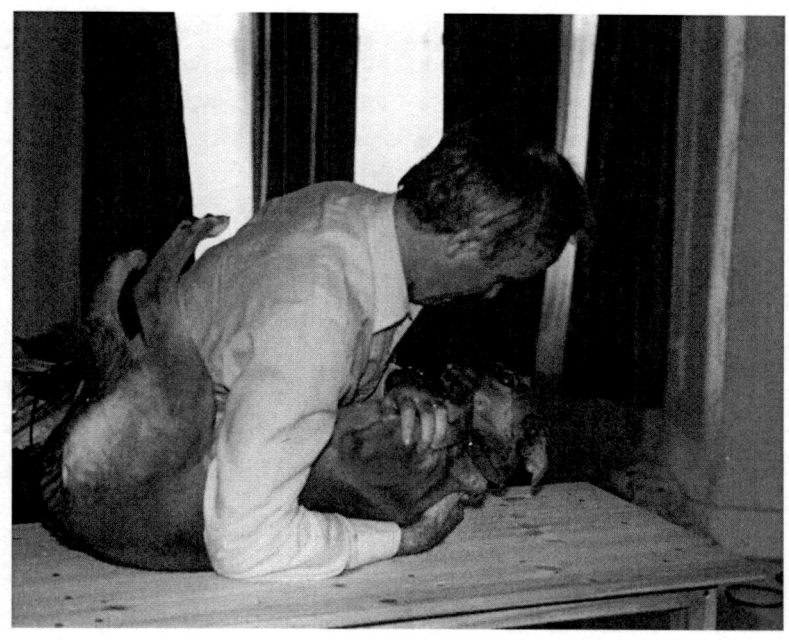

Stephan Pirie had a rather unexpected patient which called for the dog technique!

the M.O.C. We negotiated over many months for the house next door to the school, as well as other properties in the vicinity – but to no avail. There was nothing else for it, we had to build in our own grounds. Plans were drawn up for osteopathy's first custom built clinic, and this was my cue to talk to the bank as we could not rely on fundraising alone. Over the years I had a policy of keeping in close touch with the bank manager by way of regular meetings. I would update him with news of our achievements, details of our plans and the reasons for them. For some years we even had a bank manager as a trustee. It's a shame that an ongoing working relationship with the manager no longer exists in the same way in today's banking world.

Concurrent with all these events, we had formally requested inspection by the G.C. and R.O., and there was a flurry of activity preparing all the paperwork. The inspectorate attended from 7th–11th June 1982 at the end of which we were told that we had passed 'most satisfactorily' although the actual announcement was not made by the Register until 1983. Another big step forward had been taken towards the unity of the profession.

Within osteopathy there was a move towards developing formal academic structures in line with other healthcare professions such as nursing, physiotherapy, podiatry etc. There were some – and Tom was one, initially – who were against degree status, but we could not remain aloof from this trend – and survive. The profession was beginning also to look afresh at the possibility of legislation. Things were on the move – and so was our expansion programme.

Over the summer of 1983, the clinic was built – on time and on budget. Its official opening was celebrated the following spring by which time we had also completed the extension to the main lecture hall – the latter having been achieved as a result of fundraising including a generous donation from Genesis.

The official opening of our new purpose-built tutorial clinic on 19th May 1984 was performed by Dr R.H. Bannerman, World Health Organization, who came over from Geneva especially for the occasion. There were over 200 guests including the Mayor and Mayoress of Maidstone and, underlining our strong French connections, the Deputy Mayor and Mayoress of Beauvais, Maidstone's twin town. The osteopathic and medical professions were of course well represented including colleagues from France, Belgium and Holland.

By this time Ann Carroll M.B.E., M.Ed. was working with us. Miss Carroll was a retired headmistress who lived near the school. Her initial involvement was on a voluntary part-time

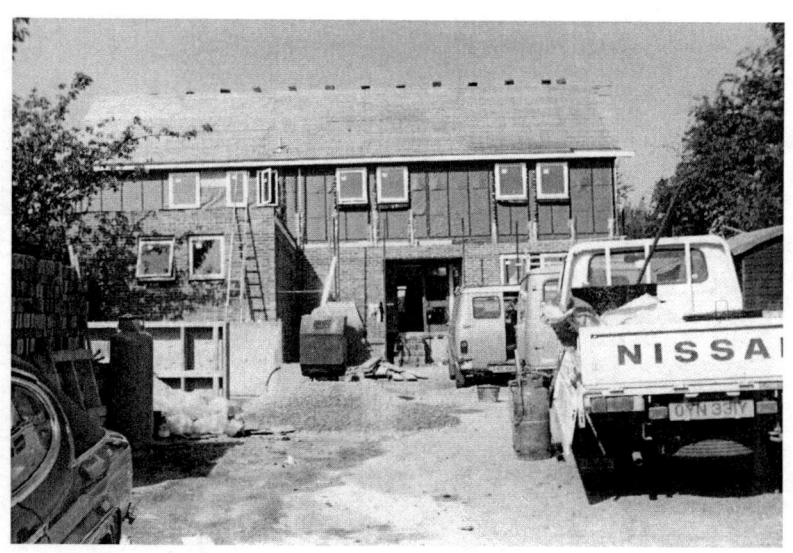

The building of the clinic at 104 Tonbridge Road

basis helping in the library. Under her direction the Library and Resource Centre was hugely improved. Eventually, she became our Education Consultant and was the school's representative on the G.C. and R.O. Standing Education Committee.

In 1982 a three-year postgraduate course for registered medical practitioners in osteopathic medicine was introduced at the Université de Paris-Nord, Bobigny. The faculty was drawn from our E.E.O. French-speaking lecturers, which was considered to be an important development. In March 1985, some 80 of the French doctors attended a three-day seminar at the E.S.O. with the object of having direct academic and social contact with the lecturers of the full-time E.S.O. course. The seminar was so successful that it became an annual event complementing the university's programme. Coinciding with the seminar was the official opening of the new garden classroom carried out by Dr Didier Feltesse, Head of Department of Osteopathic Medicine at the university.

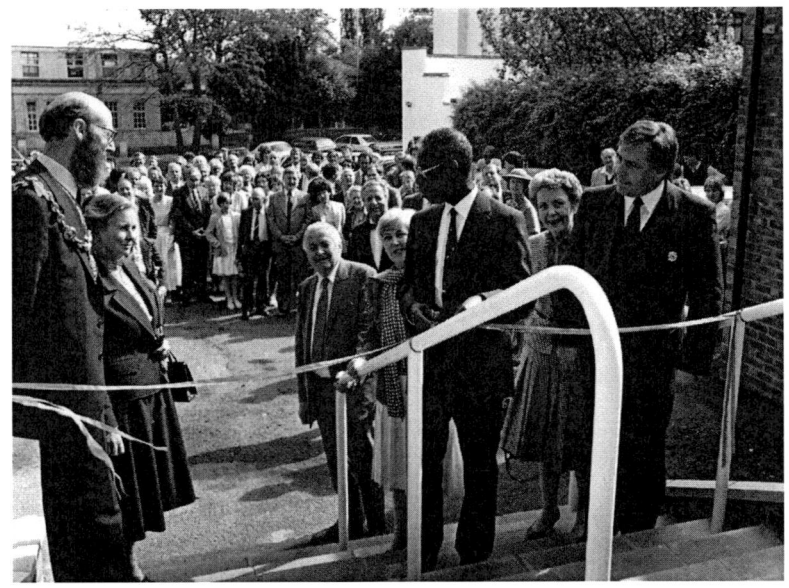

Dr R.H. Bannerman from the World Health Organization seen here cutting the ribbon to officially open the new clinic building

In 1985 I had been involved in osteopathy for 25 years. Staff and students got together and organised a delightful surprise party for me – and this was followed by a presentation from the Society of Osteopaths. I felt very spoilt!

In spite of all the good things that were happening around this time we had to cope with a mega problem – dry rot! Who was it who said, 'About the time we think we can make ends meet, somebody moves the ends!' When we bought 104 Tonbridge Road, the surveyor's report indicated that there was rot present. We obtained three quotations from specialist firms, and chose the one recommended by the surveyor who had used them previously with complete satisfaction. A year or so later I heard on the news that the company had gone into liquidation. When the dry rot was discovered, the 30-year guarantee we had on file was worthless. The builders moved in and the whole of the

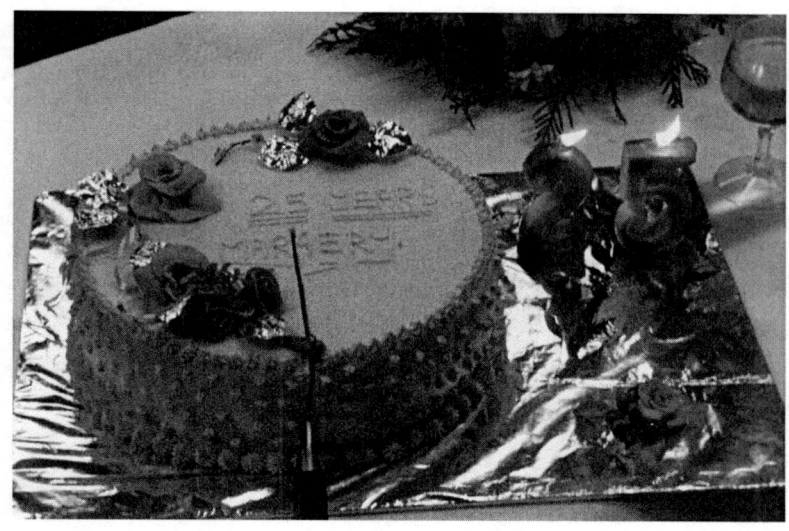

25 years in osteopathy

front of the building had to be gutted. I remember standing near the front door looking up through two floors and seeing the sky. This meant moving ourselves into those areas not affected. In spite of cramped conditions, dust and noise, not one lecture was cancelled. The students and staff were brilliant. There was so much to complain about – but nobody did. With such great support and careful budgeting we were back on track by the following year.

The clinic was proving to be a great success and to everyone's joy it was growing steadily. Faculty members and admin staff were supportive of the students, the students were supportive of each other and once they were in the clinic, a caring attitude towards the patients was always evident. In the process of providing the essential clinical experience for students, the clinic also served the community by providing treatment for people of limited means. Our policy was that nobody was ever turned away for lack of funds.

Of course there could be some ripples on the water from time to time. There were even occasions when I felt I was running a kindergarten, whilst at others it seemed more like a living soap opera! *Most* of the time however there was a happy, positive atmosphere; visitors to the school always remarked on it, and there was a never-ending stream of visitors – colleagues from all over the world used to pop in to see what the E.S.O. was all about. With the passage of time, we gained quite a reputation for our hospitality and at suitable moments there was always a bottle of wine handy – echoing our French roots. Good habits tend to linger!

Demand for places in the school was increasing every year. By the end of the 1980s we were dealing with around 1,000 enquiries a year which would result in perhaps 150 plus firm applications. Our capacity for new first years was around 25. Space problems were once again on the horizon. Earlier in the 1980s we made a mistake one year by accepting 63 first years on the Cours Francophone, which meant dividing them into two groups. It was a timetabling nightmare and we decided that for the future quality was far more important than quantity.

Any amount of hard work and long hours has never bothered me, having been blessed with more energy than most, but dealing with difficult people I did find stressful. It always seemed to fall to me to hire, fire and discipline. 'Disciplining', whether a student or staff member, was my least favourite job. However, on one of the rare occasions when it was necessary, it turned out to be hilarious. I was sitting behind my desk trying to make clear that a particular situation could not continue. The person (who shall be nameless) refused to recognise the error of his ways. To reinforce the importance of what I was saying, I stood up intending to walk round to the other side of my desk and face him at close quarters. As luck would have it, the zips on the insides of the knee-high boots I was wearing locked together so that when I went to take a step, I fell flat on my face. Neither of us could stop laughing. Talk about an icebreaker! It is amazing how many problems can be solved with a little humour, even if it is unplanned.

Whilst on the topic of interviewing, I have been surprised by the number of graduates who, over the years, have told me how clearly they remember their first interview with me. I confess I cannot remember them all but there are a few amusing interviews I do recall that are worth sharing. On one occasion there was a very large woman, who sat in the rather small armchair next to my desk. The interview had gone well but when she stood up to leave, the armchair was still attached to her bottom. Quickly I stood up and wrenched it off – embarrassing all round!

Then there was the man I had spoken to on the telephone. He had a big, deep voice but when he arrived, to my surprise, he was only about four foot tall (or short depending on how you look at it) one of the few people I have ever towered over.

Another interview I shall never forget was when two executive gentlemen from the electricity suppliers came along to advise me on some heating problems. As it happened, that day there were cranial lectures and I had handed the lecturer some finger cots for mouth work. One got left behind and was sitting on my desk. The two men sat opposite me and I was suddenly aware that one of them had seen the finger cot. He was unable to hide the thoughts that were clearly racing through his mind and every other sentence his eyes kept returning to the finger cot. Was it – or wasn't it?

Then there was the prospective student who, obviously, was 'on something'. There was a good minute's delay between my questions and his answers. Another applicant who comes to mind told me he had just returned from a week on retreat, meditating. He was so 'spaced out' during the interview that he nearly fell off his chair. I just caught him in time.

By the mid '80s more and more students were receiving discretionary awards from local education authorities but we had to wait a bit longer for the Inner London Education Authority.

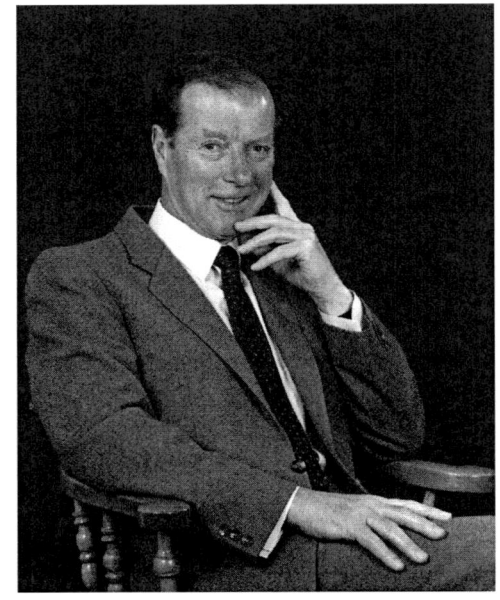

Peter Blagrave

In July 1987 Tom retired as principal but took the title of Principal Emeritus and remained president of the school's sponsoring company O.E. & R. Ltd. He continued to be involved in various ways and used to ring me regularly to keep up to date with everything that was going on.

At the beginning of the academic year 1987/88 Peter Blagrave took over as principal of the full-time side of the school whilst Barrie Savory headed the Cours Francophone. Unfortunately, in January 1988, Peter fell ill with a serious heart problem and had to relinquish his post.

Academic session 1988/89 saw Barrie Savory as overall principal of the school. As with previous principals, due to the

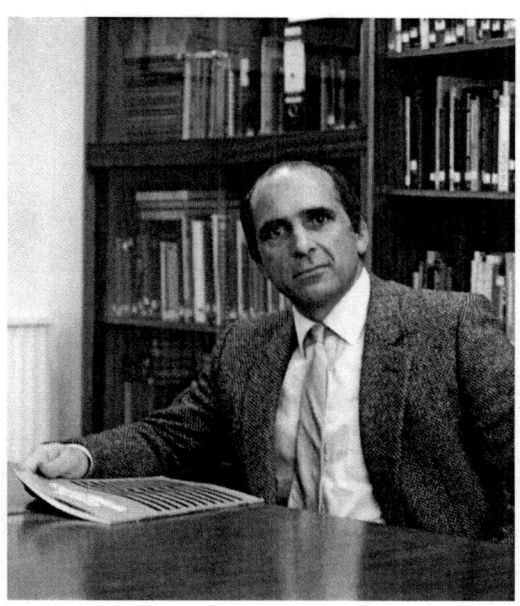

Barrie Savory

school's financial constraints it was a one day a week job, plus any additional lecturing and school commitments.

Barrie and I worked well together, and having a similar sense of humour helped us get through the difficult patches. In spite of the time restrictions, we achieved a lot during the following few years, aided greatly in all things academic by the addition of Dr Paula Fletcher Bsc PhD P.G.C.E. who joined us in September 1989. Paula was already familiar with the world of osteopathy as she had been education officer with the G.C. and R.O. for a couple of years. I remember when she first started with us, building work was in progress and there was so little available space, she almost had to work standing up! By October, happily, the large first floor extension was finished and she had her own office, as well as a lot more space for the support staff.

As part of the work towards legislation a survey of osteopathic education in the U.K. was carried out by the British Accreditation Council. The Inspectorate's three day visit to the E.S.O. was in February 1988. The subsequent report on the school was 'most satisfactory'. Later that year we had the G.C.

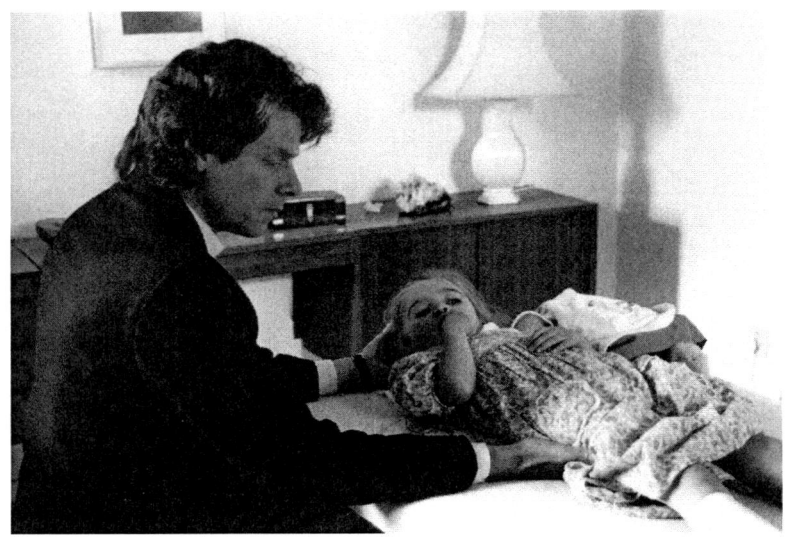

Stuart Korth treating a young patient in the children's clinic

and R.O.'s quinquennial inspection as well, which reconfirmed our accreditation status. There is such a lot of time and effort involved in preparing the paperwork for inspections but, perversely perhaps, I really enjoyed them. It was a great stimulus to reassess and to go on improving every aspect of our operation.

Up until this time the school's postgraduate activities had taken place in close collaboration with the Society of Osteopaths but now the time had come for the school to set up its own Department of Postgraduate Studies which we launched in May 1989. We held a gala three-day conference in the French language under the title of Premières Rencontres Maidstoniennes. The reason for the title was that for our French-speaking colleagues, Maidstone was synonymous with osteopathy. The conference proved to be a great success – academically and socially – and from the letters received following the event the consensus of opinion seemed to be 'More please.'

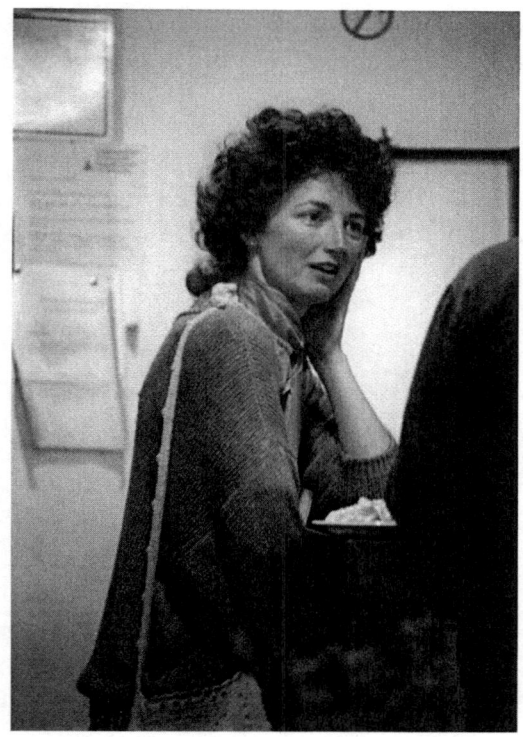

Sue Turner

In 1989 we started a children's clinic as an integral part of our teaching clinic. It was under the direction of Stuart Korth, widely regarded as the most experienced children's osteopath in the country. Treatment was offered for children from babies to young teenagers, as well as pre- and post-natal osteopathic care. The team of tutors was headed by Sue Turner.

The following year Stuart Korth approached us about some ideas he had for creating a children's institute offering treatment, training, postgraduate work and research. We were very enthusiastic about his proposals but in the end Stuart decided to go it alone and form a separate registered charity called the Osteopathic Centre for Children. From humble beginnings – a Saturday clinic held at the Royal London Homoeopathic Hospital in Great Ormond Street, London – the O.C.C. grew and flourished, eventually having its own premises – and doing wonderful work.

Sue Turner did a great job continuing to run the Children's Clinic over many years, in addition to lecturing. Indeed in the

1980s there was a considerable number of faculty members who made most praiseworthy sacrifices in order to help get the school established.

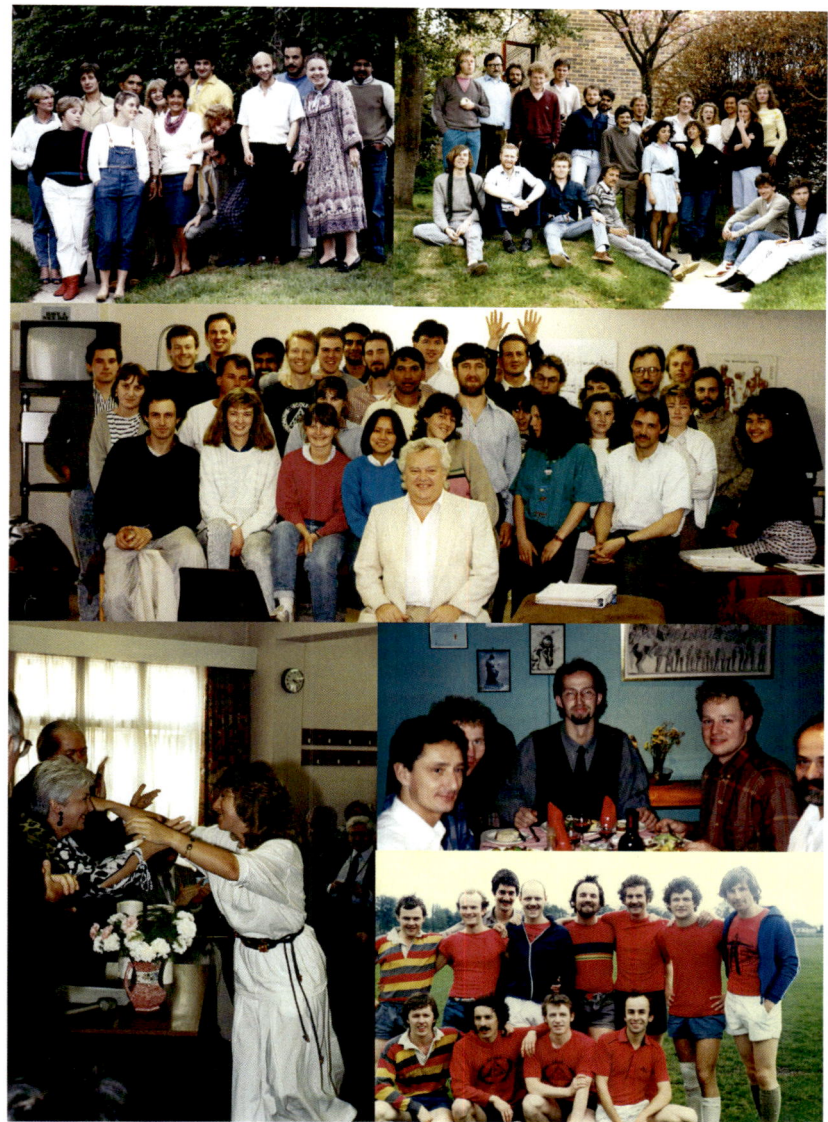

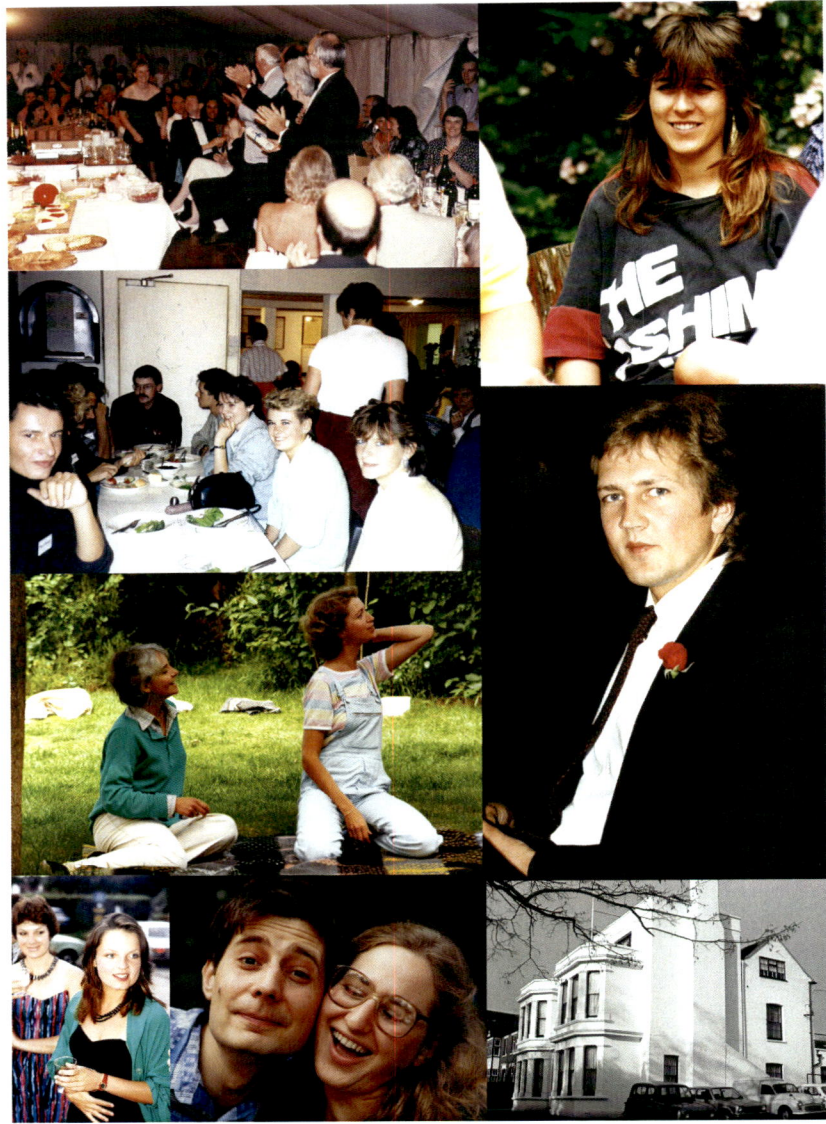

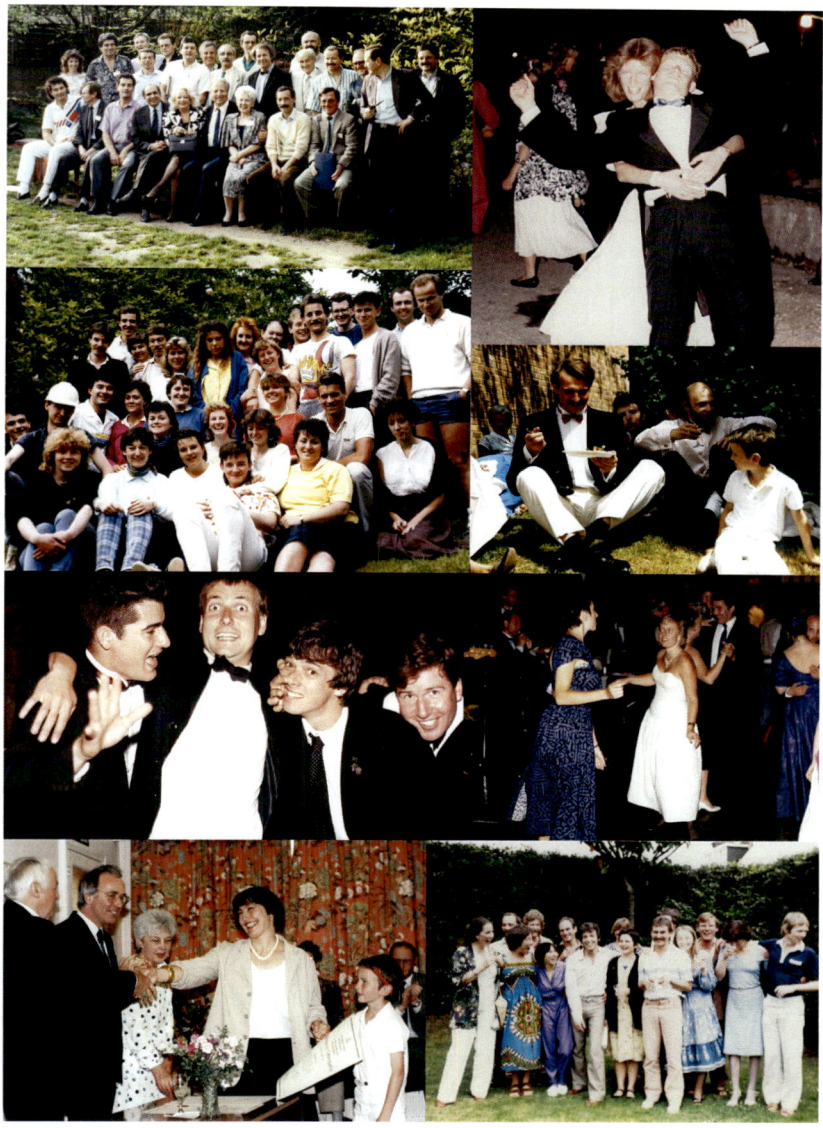

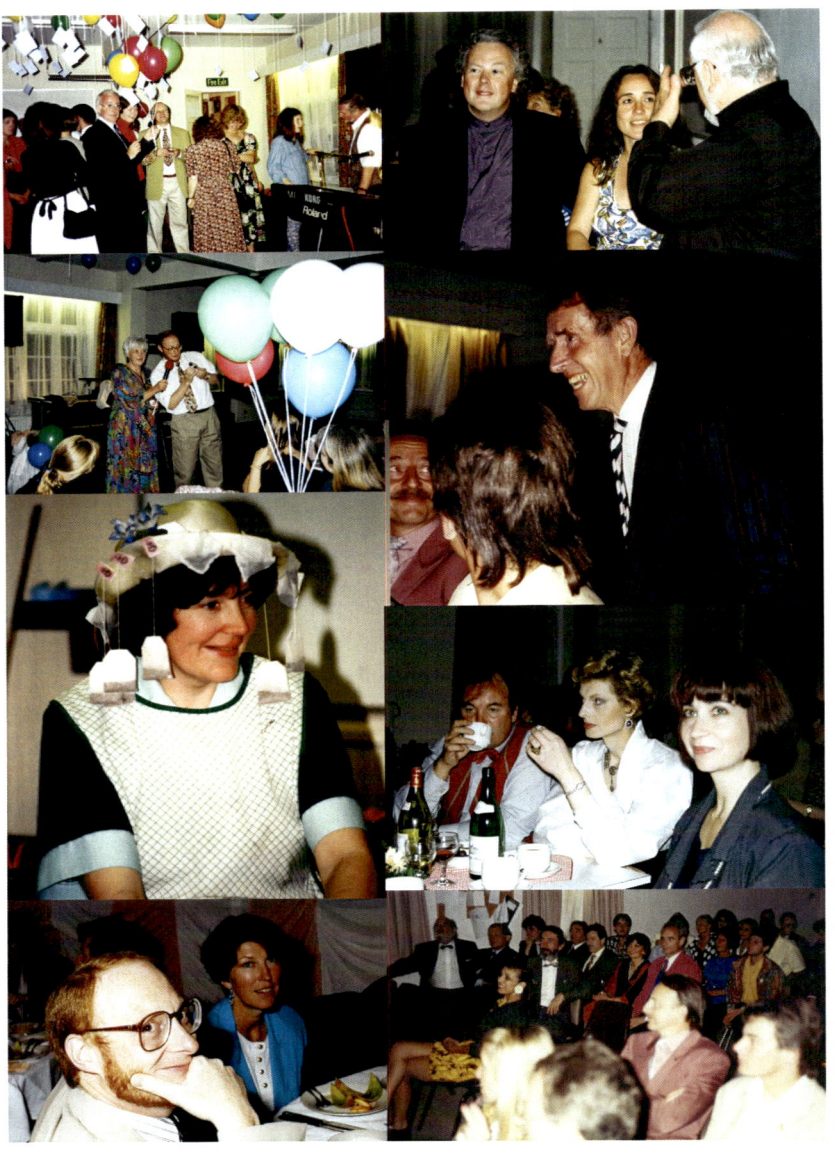

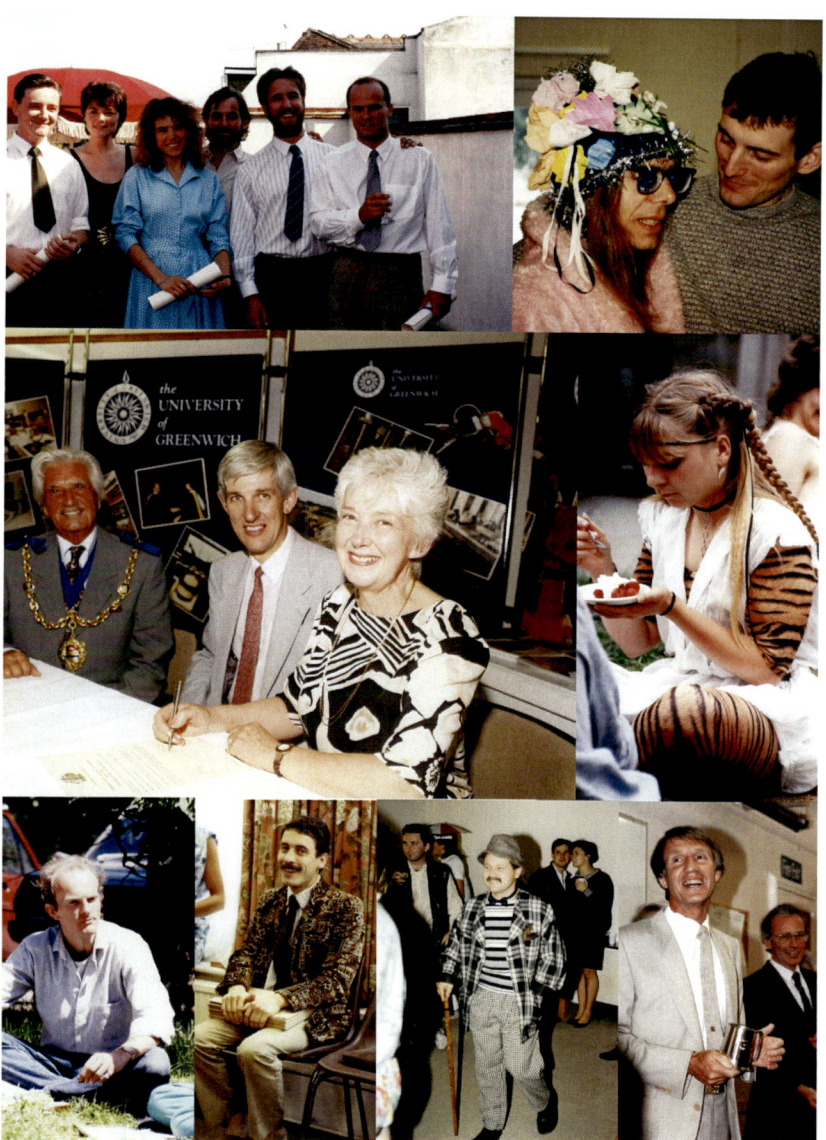

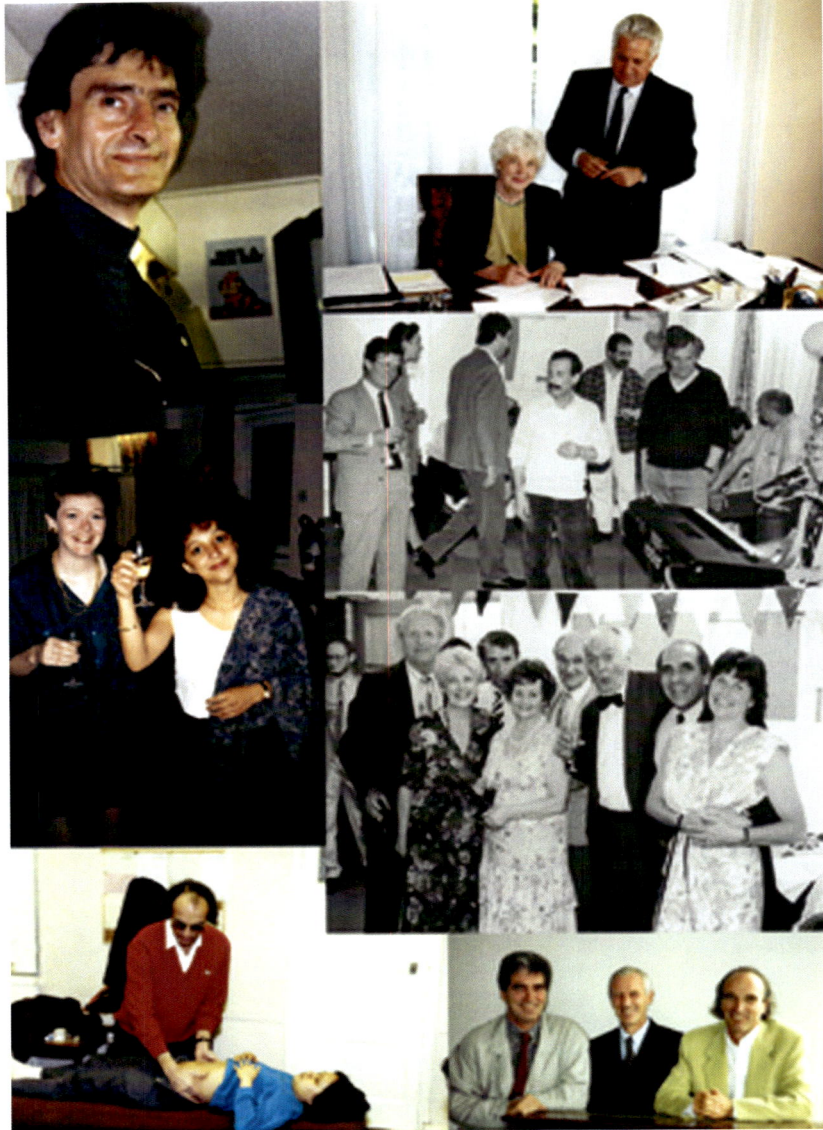

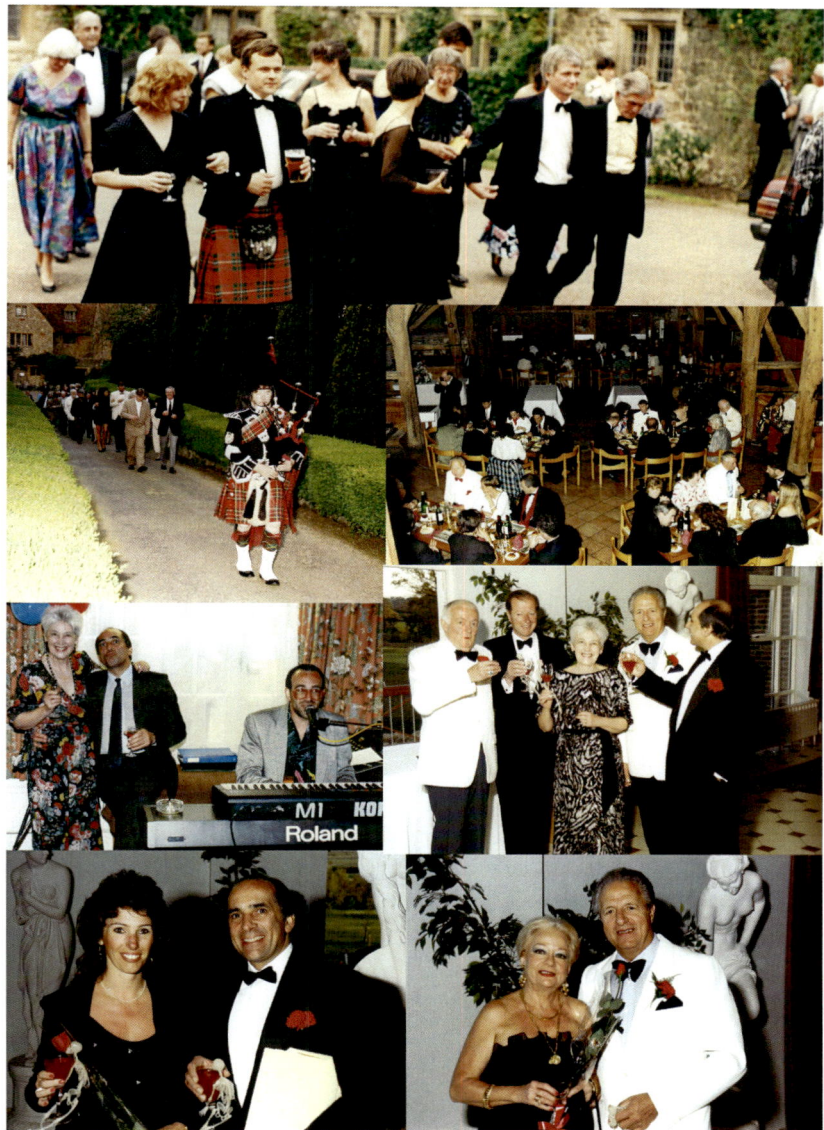

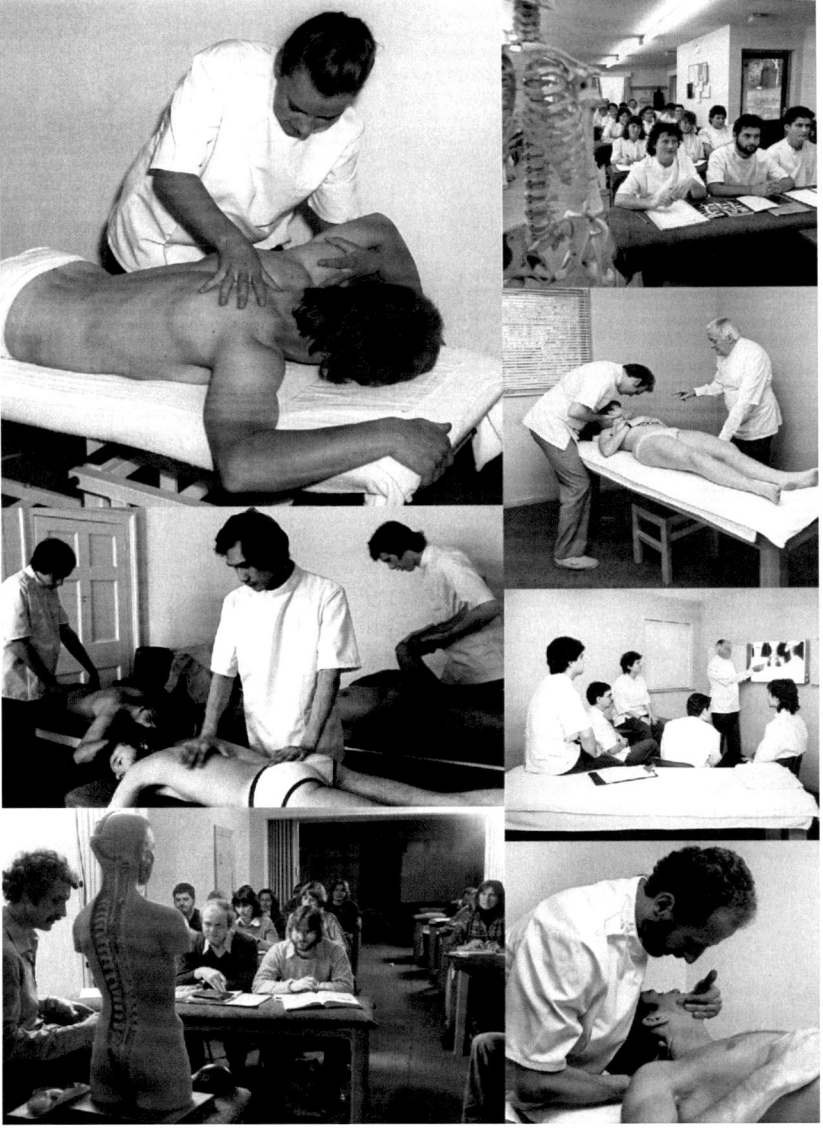

Chapter Ten

E.E.O. Developments and International Academic Links

> *'A gem cannot be polished without friction,*
> *nor man perfected without trials'*
> — Chinese Proverb

Running the E.E.O. and the E.S.O. was like running two different schools. They were poles apart in terms of administration, finance, the personalities involved, and the problems; but the teaching material was the same, although differently arranged. There is no doubt that the cross fertilisation between the E.E.O. and the E.S.O. was an important contribution to the richness of the school's osteopathy. The E.E.O. course, over the years, was called variously 'postgraduate', 'part time', 'tutorial' and finally 'Cours Francophone' and to avoid confusion I will use the latter term in this chapter.

As time went on our Belgian and French colleagues were keen to add extra seminars in their respective countries and they began to look for suitable venues. They wanted to set themselves up as branches of the school and Tom was quite keen to go along with their ideas but I was not at all enthusiastic, as I could foresee problems.

However, the course was restructured to allow for the additional seminars, in Lyon and Wégimont, to be introduced. This arrangement worked well initially but after a while our auditors and the trustees began to question the legality, in view of our charitable status, of setting up French and Belgian branches. We sought the advice of our solicitors and it was confirmed that branches could not function autonomously in the name of the school; they had to be disbanded. Henceforth the 'branch managers', Ange Castejon and Pierre Corriat, would be known as 'Delegate Representatives' of the E.E.O. School bank accounts were opened in France and Belgium and all financial transactions were to be subject to audit in the usual way by the School's auditors in the UK. This proved to be easier said than done!

In June 1980 S.B.O. and R.T.M, the Belgian osteopathic society, all members of which were graduates of the E.E.O., organised a European Osteopathic Congress attended by 600 delegates. In the years ahead they repeated their success by hosting several other major conferences. For a relatively small organisation our Belgian colleagues, headed by Pierre Corriat, were very active and constantly achieving. They also started their own printing set-up producing, for example, six volumes of the E.E.O. lecturers' courses, superbly illustrated by one of the students, Godeliève Struyf-Denys – and other osteopathic books followed.

In September 1981 the Belgians succeeded in opening an osteopathic clinic in Brussels. At the official ceremony something happened which I have never forgotten – and it still makes me smile. Pierre Corriat was addressing the guests and I happened to be standing in the front row. He was saying that there were key people in osteopathy they wished to honour by naming various rooms in the clinic after them. For example there was the Tom Dummer room, the Colin Dove room, the Professor John Upledger room – and others I cannot remember. Then with a look of 'oops' on his face when he looked at me Pierre added quickly – and we are naming the basement after Margery Bloomfield. It amused me so much I don't know how I controlled my laughter. Well, at least it wasn't the loo that was named after me!

On the occasion of one of the Belgian conferences I have fond memories of a spontaneous osteopathic jazz happening. A group of us were relaxing in the music bar of our hotel but there was no band and no other customers. Suddenly it happened – Tom Dummer and John Upledger on pianos, Fred Mitchell on double bass and Ange Castejon tap dancing. A pity I did not have my camera with me.

Another memory of a very different kind has just sprung to mind. We were due to attend an osteopathic meeting in Paris in October – the exact date of which coincided with the annual motor show. It proved to be impossible to find hotel accommodation so in the end I rang one of the French students and asked for help. When he rang back to say he had found somewhere I thought he sounded almost apologetic. The hotel was in a back street on the left bank. On arrival Robert asked for a bottle of Perrier water to be sent up. 'Not champagne Monsieur?' asked the concierge. When we got to our room we realised the significance of his question. This was a 'studio à l'heure' hotel. The décor was bright pink and black with mirrors covering the ceiling and two of the walls. The breakfast was good too…

Enough of frivolity.

The Cours Francophone problems continued unabated. Tom was tiring of the endless bickering and announced that he wished to relinquish all responsibility for the Cours Francophone. Ange Castejon was appointed to replace him but Tom retained the principalship of the full-time side. Our colleagues across the Channel showed a total lack of understanding about the school's charitable status – no matter how many times we tried to explain it. In addition the school's auditors were exasperated by their inadequate financial records and reluctance to provide more information when requested. The situation was reaching fever pitch.

In July 1985 when all concerned were present for the end of year exams, I came up with a possible solution and called everyone into my office for a frank discussion. In spite of all the differences, we shared the common ideal of providing the best possible training in osteopathy which seemed to me an excellent basis on which we could build. My suggestion was that we should separate England, France and Belgium financially and administratively but *not* academically. The idea was that they should set up an organisation in France and another in Belgium to undertake the *partial* training of the French-speaking students enrolled in the E.E.O. This met with approval and I agreed to clear these proposed plans with our solicitors.

Verbal agreement was one thing, action was quite another. It turned out that, on reflection, they wanted everything to remain as it had been and so defiantly continued to organise seminars in Belgium and France in the name of the school – and did nothing about setting up the independent organisations. The situation was getting worse by the minute when, out of the blue, came some good news – a mea culpa letter from our French representative. Having been friends with Ange for over a quarter of a century it was a great relief that the rift was over. Our Belgian colleagues however remained intransigent. There is no point in going into details, it is all water under the bridge but I did find it sad that Pierre, who had done so much excellent work for osteopathy in Belgium, should now be attacking the school with such vehemence. I always suspected there was a hidden agenda but whatever the motive things came to a head in December 1986 when our Belgian representative sent a scurrilous dossier to every E.E.O. student and lecturer.

Enough was enough – firm action was called for and we announced that in future *all* seminars would be held in Maidstone. End of story. We appointed Barrie Savory as Director of the Cours Francophone. Fortunately, the vast majority of the students 'saw through' the attack on the E.E.O. and responded with a great display of loyalty to the school. When the next seminar was held in Maidstone, it was declared the 'best ever'. Peace had returned. We had weathered yet another storm. In steering the school through its various difficulties, I found it was essential to keep one's nerve *and* one's sense of humour. I must admit that this particular storm had been tedious, and I was grateful for the support I received in the background from one of the French students. His name was Renzo Molinari – more anon.

Whenever I meet up with Barrie Savory, we usually reminisce about the school. There is one story which might amuse because it still amuses us when we recall it. We had been in one of those heated meetings with French-speaking colleagues, at the end of which they had left the office but Barrie and I went on discussing the pros and cons of the situation. After some ten minutes or so, we suddenly realised we were still speaking French to each other!

By 1986 osteopathic schools were mushrooming in France and beginning elsewhere in Europe as well. In view of this we decided it was time to run down the Cours Francophone over the next six years by not accepting any more new first-year students. Our task had come to an end.

In November 1986 at a meeting of the Association Française des Ostéopathes, who were all graduates of the E.E.O., it was decided unanimously that the spirit and teaching of the E.E.O. had to continue in France. A meeting was arranged for January 1987 in Paris. The outcome was that the Collège International d'Ostéopathie (C.I.D.O.) was founded with the full blessing and cooperation of the E.E.O. It was to be based in St. Etienne and would offer a seminar-based course over six years, virtually identical to the E.E.O.'s Cours Francophone, but administratively and financially separate. To maintain the close connection with the 'Mother School' there would be one seminar per year held in Maidstone for each class of the six-year course, thus giving them the benefit of the English faculty. In addition the E.E.O. accepted to participate in the examinations, which would be held in Maidstone.

The three colleagues with whom Barrie Savory, Robert and myself met in Paris were to become the three Directeurs of C.I.D.O. Jean-Pierre Barral (académique) Patrick Féval (administratif) and Jacques Descotes (relations extérieures.) This was the beginning of another important chapter in the history of the school.

I have sometimes been asked what happened to the French osteopaths after they qualified. Well, those who were undeterred by the possibility of a 'procés' for the illegal practice of medicine simply closed their physiotherapy practices, and started afresh as osteopaths. Others, who were more cautious, practised under cover of their physiotherapy diplomas. A few went on to qualify in medicine, some of them returning to the E.E.O. to lecture. There were also some who, for a variety of reasons, did not practise osteopathy at all, even though they had qualified. Of course the whole question of 'fines' was a big consideration and some osteopaths were hit harder than others. As time went on things improved slightly. There were even some judges who would make only a nominal one franc fine.

When we were approached about cooperating with the Université de Paris-Nord, Bobigny (see previous chapter), we were at first a little hesitant, given the legal situation in France at the time. On balance we felt it would be better to be involved and be sure of the quality of the teaching than stand aside from something that was going to happen anyway. It came about as a result of the Doyen of the Faculty of Medicine going to an osteopath for treatment – and the osteopath was a graduate of the E.E.O. Our academic link with the Bobigny doctors was a very positive experience. With the passage of time there were several of them who joined the E.E.O. faculty, which brought them to Maidstone on a regular basis. Dr Didier Feltesse, for example, was a frequent visitor and, a little later, Dr Eric Thévenet of whom more in the next chapter.

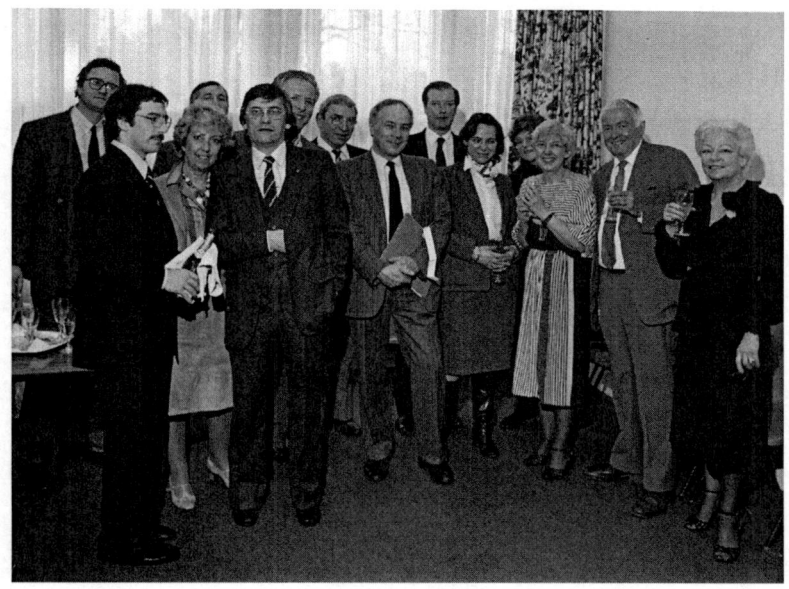

Reception at the school to welcome the Doyen of the Faculty of Medicine, University of Paris-Nord, Bobigny.

A national osteopathic examination was introduced in Belgium. This necessitated a meeting with representatives of the Belgian osteopathic society on 5th August 1989. Happily, no reference was made to the major problems of the past. The meeting was cordial and it was agreed that the E.E.O. would have a representative present whenever our students were examined. Of equal importance it was agreed that in the interests of European osteopathy we would remain in touch.

In July 1992 the last graduates of our Cours Francophone received their diplomas at a Gala Supper Party held at the school, marking the end of yet another era. To coincide with the presentation of diplomas we organised a conference in the French language under the title of 'L'homme Total' and invited three of the school's earliest graduates to lecture.

Among the final E.E.O. graduates was the group from Guadeloupe. Initially contact had been made with them by Ange Castejon and Fernand-Paul Berthenet who had visited the island. Soon we had set up a course over six years with E.E.O. lecturers going to Guadeloupe (without any reluctance at all need I add!) and the group making regular visits to Maidstone. They brought the sunshine with them each time and everyone enjoyed having them around. Typically they also brought the ingredients for an end-of-the-day Caribbean cocktail as well.

There was another island group we had the pleasure of training. Some of our E.E.O. lecturers had been visiting Île de la Réunion and had been invited to deliver some lectures on osteopathy to a group of physiotherapists. After a while they wished to have a more structured course. An academic link was established with the school and we were able to adapt the Cours Francophone to their needs.

In addition to C.I.D.O., we had an arrangement with another French school – Collège Ostéopathique Français in Paris. It too had been started by graduates of the E.E.O. Dr André Ratio who, after graduating, went on to study medicine and Renzo Molinari who became the director of C.O.F.

Yet another graduate, Roland Lorillieux, asked for our help in getting a school set up in Spain. Italy also wanted academic links with us through a graduate of the full-time course, Alfonso Mandara. Sweden too sought our help through Bengt Elmstrom, an early E.S.O. graduate, with Skandinaviska Osteopatskolan.

In autumn 1996, some Belgian colleagues started a school called Collège Belge d'Ostéopathie (C.B.O.) and they wanted to renew links with the E.E.O. It was very pleasing to be back working with them again.

There were indeed many requests from graduates in Europe and beyond seeking our help to start schools or develop programmes. Our international policy, initially, had been to establish academic links *only* with E.E.O./E.S.O. graduates in other countries, who were aspiring to start serious training establishments. Our reasoning was that we knew their standards and we knew them as people, and this was a positive basis for helping them achieve their objectives. However in a changing osteopathic world it was time to widen the net.

In 1996 we hosted a seminar for students of the Austrian school, Wiener Schule für Osteopathie. In the same year a series of three postgraduate seminars, two in Maidstone and one in Switzerland, was arranged for the Association Suisse des Ostéopathes. Discussions began regarding future collaboration with both organisations.

In March 1996 I asked my vice-principal, then Renzo Molinari, to represent the school at the American Osteopathic Association conference in Atlanta. There he met two Russian delegates who were interested in the setting up of an osteopathic course. It was arranged that they would make a trip to Maidstone. Renzo and I had in-depth discussions with them, out of which came our working relationship with the Academy of Child Development in St. Petersburg. We sent our lecturers to Russia at regular intervals and they came to us in the summer for an intensive two-week seminar. The Russian group was made up of physicians, surgeons, medical specialists and paramedicals. It would be difficult to find more enthusiastic and appreciative students – and this is still the case 13 years later! Our Russian friends are so rewarding to teach and great fun socially as well.

This brief summary of our international activities covers the period up to my retirement in September 1997. My successor built on this and spread the influence of the school far and wide, as will be recounted in the next chapter.

Chapter Eleven

European School of Osteopathy

> *'If it can be done, it should be done now.
> If it is impossible, it may take a little time.'*
> — Admiral Richard Kempenfelt

ALL THE OTHER decades had been extremely busy but the 1990s were even more action packed – and full of achievements. We were thinking seriously now about degree status, and the search for the right partner began.

There was much enthusiasm amongst certain faculty members to have our first postgraduate seminar in English, having launched the department the year before with a successful P.G. seminar in French. Jeremy Gilbey, Sue Turner, Joyce Vetterlein, Jim Sumerfield and others were bursting with ideas for possible programmes. On one of her trips to the U.S.A., Sue Turner had met Dr Frank Willard, distinguished American anatomist who, at the time, was Associate Professor of Anatomy and Director of Medical Curriculum at the University of New England College of Osteopathic Medicine. Barrie Savory and I agreed this would be an excellent choice and the invitation was issued for March 1990. Frank Willard's thought-provoking style of presentation was a huge success – and other visits followed. Then in 1992 I asked Frank if he would consider joining the faculty of the E.S.O. He agreed and I am pleased to say that to this day he continues to make regular visits to the school. I have often wondered how many thousands of miles he has travelled on our behalf. Undergraduate and postgraduate students, as well as those involved in our international connections, have all benefited enormously from Frank Williard's inspiring and stimulating anatomy lectures as well as the presentations of his dissection work at the University.

Our philosophy for postgraduate events was to make them not only relevant and interesting but an enjoyable social occasion as well. To this end I made sure that there were flowers everywhere, a warm welcome, a special lunch and a long enough break to allow people to mix and chat. Participants included graduates of all the schools as well as some local doctors and health professionals, which provided useful bridge-building opportunities. This must have been the right policy because most programmes were a sell-out, and some even had a waiting list.

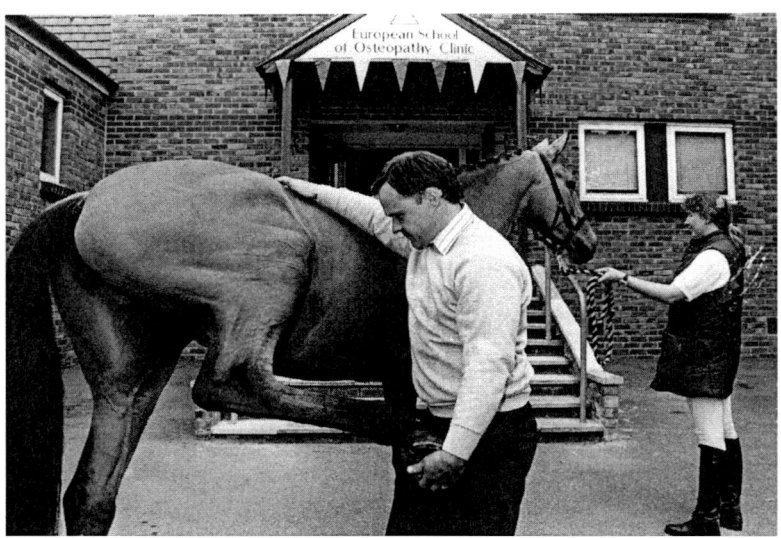

Stuart MacGregor treating a horse

In December 1990 it was 25 years since the school had relocated to England, which we felt was worthy of a big celebration, but December was not the right month for all the ideas I had running around in my head. We settled for the first weekend in June 1991. We started with a golf tournament on the Friday for those so inclined followed by two days of lectures in both English and French covering a wide range of topics including practical demonstrations of animal osteopathy.

In mentioning animal osteopathy I am reminded that when Stuart MacGregor was a student he asked if he could write his final year dissertation on osteopathy and the horse. We thought about that request for some days but finally agreed. It turned out to be the most frequently requested dissertation in the library. Subsequently, a number of other students and graduates gravitated towards animal osteopathy – and I am delighted to see that trend has continued and expanded.

Back to the 25th anniversary, a celebration supper party was held on the Saturday evening at Nettlestead Place, a medieval manor house set in 12 acres of garden. Guests were piped in by a Scottish piper, sipped cocktails on the terrace to the sounds of a Caribbean steel band and then had supper and dancing in a marquee with jazz band and a barbershop quintet for entertainment. Leeds Castle was the venue for the Sunday evening Gala Dinner Dance with the talented Steve McKie providing music and entertainment. We welcomed 220 guests from all around the world who proclaimed it 'a truly memorable event'.

Looking back I guess the school was something of a party animal – we seemed to have a lot of them! Was it something to do with our French origin? (Or was it just that Margery liked organizing such events – and I still do!) Whatever the occasion I always made sure that it was cost effective as it was important that our international get-togethers paid for themselves. I remain convinced that the feel-good factor engendered by osteopathic gatherings is of real value for both the school and the profession.

On 28th September 1991 there was another gathering, this time in France, to celebrate the official opening of the Collège International d'Ostéopathie headquarters in St. Etienne. The splendid property, formerly a family dwelling house, provided accommodation for the administrative offices and a large classroom block had been built in the garden.

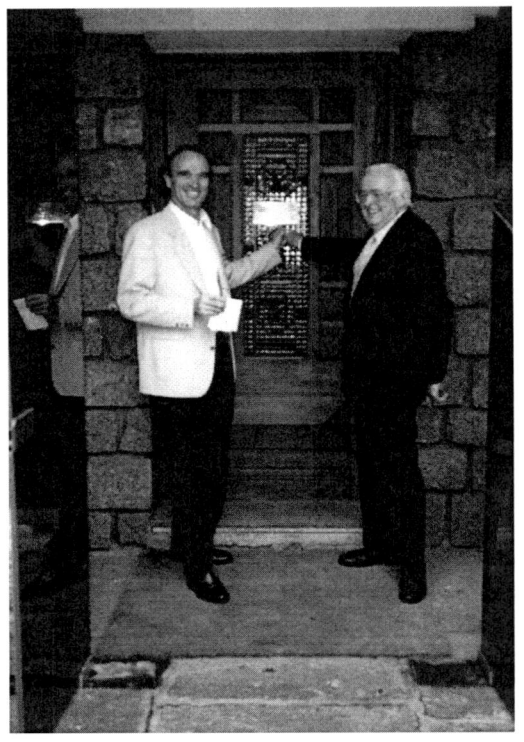

Jean-Pierre Barral with Tom Dummer pointing to the plate on the front door of Maison Thomas Dummer

The building was named 'Maison Thomas Dummer'. An excellent soirée followed the inauguration ceremony.

Ever since accreditation by the G.C. and R.O., the French-speaking graduates of the Cours Francophone had expressed interest in joining the Register. Eventually so many had posed the question that we took the matter up with the G.C. and R.O. After much discussion the Register signalled its acceptance in principle of the proposal but advised that their Education Department would have to examine acceptable methods of assessment for deciding the eligibility of each candidate. In the meantime I was asked to find out how many of our graduates might wish to avail themselves of the opportunity of applying for membership. This was in June 1991. By the time the information was gathered we were moving ever nearer to legislation which meant that in the fullness of time the Register would cease to exist and be replaced by the General Osteopathic Council. So that was the end of that rather pointless exercise.

The search for the right university to take us forward to degree status was well under way, headed by Dr Paula Fletcher. There was a lot of interest in the E.S.O. but the conditions had to be favourable. We did not want to be swallowed up and lose our identity and independence. In 1991 Barrie Savory decided to relinquish his post. This was mutually regretted but he felt that a one-day-a-week principal could not meet the needs of the school as it moved towards degree status.

The board of governors agreed that the school should now have its first full-time principal and they asked me if I would consider taking on the role. At first I was reluctant as I had always felt that an osteopath should be principal, providing there was somebody suitable to look after finance and administration, plus an educationalist. One by one I was 'taken out to lunch' by board or management members who tried to persuade me to accept the role. Barrie pointed out that I had always done the job anyway, so why not have the title. Tom reminded me that nobody knew the school better than I did, including all the complexities of the international side.

Ann Carroll added her thoughts with customary firmness saying 'You are what the school needs at this moment in time. There's no debate – you must accept' – and accept I did. On 1st November 1991, I became the first woman principal of an osteopathic school and the E.S.O.'s first full-time principal.

I must admit that in the past, always having to delay decisions until matters could be discussed with the principal, was a source of considerable frustration. Now it was time for lots of action and I made a list of all the major things I wanted to help the school achieve during my term of office – in other words another of my three-to-five year plans.

The first task was to develop a new management infrastructure. Paula Fletcher's title became, more appropriately, Academic Registrar. The board agreed that I could have two vice principals. Dr Nic Rowley had been lecturing with us for some time. It had been quite a struggle to get him on the faculty, even though he wanted to join us, due to his other commitments. However, with some lateral thinking, I managed it and he became a highly valued lecturer, popular with students and staff alike. He accepted to become Vice Principal (Basic and Clinical Science). For my Vice Principal (Osteopathy) I wanted Simon Fielding. He too accepted but we were both aware that his available time was going to be limited due to the pressure of his work in taking the profession towards statutory regulation. We four formed the school's Executive Committee and we worked very well together.

To complete the new infrastructure two coordinators were appointed: Sarah Wallace to work with Nic Rowley, Gez Lamb to work with Simon Fielding and Anna Reeve to link the coordinators' work. Making a start on research Vaughan Hedley was appointed Director of Clinical Research. In the clinic Peter Blagrave, who was working with us again, was Clinic Director with Jill Mew as his deputy as well as the Examinations Co-ordinator. On the French side of the School, Marilia Vasquet was appointed Directrice d'Etudes Francophones. With this capable team all now in post and excellent support staff, it was time to take a long hard look at curriculum development. We needed a fresh creative approach to prepare us for degree status – and not only a BSc Hons, I wanted us to go for an MSc as well.

Also on my 'To Do' list was to establish a graduates' club and introduce a printed news magazine. The Society of Osteopaths was now defunct so we offered to take it over and turn it into the School's alumni society. It was renamed European Society of Osteopaths (E.S.O.) loosely translated as Entente

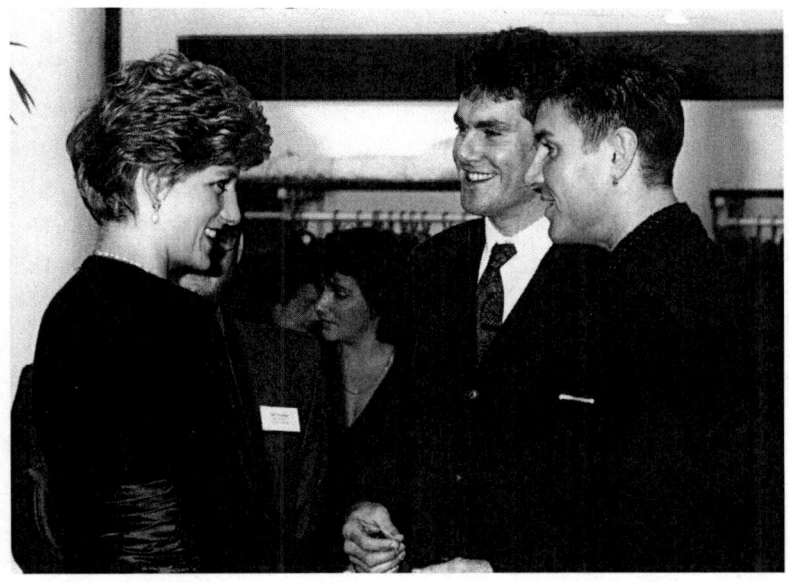

Princess Diana meeting Simon le Bon, the Duran Duran star, with his brother Jonathan who was a student at the E.S.O. at the G.C. & R.O. Reception

Européenne des Ostéopathes (E.E.O.) thus keeping the same initials.

In the Spring of 1992 we launched the E.S.O./E.E.O. Bulletin, printed in both English and French in such a way that both languages were of equal importance – which was my way of keeping graduates happy, as there had always been a competitive edge between the two sides of the school. The aim of course was to keep everyone in touch with the school, with each other and with developments within the profession. It was distributed worldwide and was most favourably received. Editing the Bulletin was one of my favourite jobs.

There were several other items on my list including staff development, increasing international and postgraduate activities, fundraising, etc. but by far the greatest challenge was going to be finding larger premises – and the search began in earnest.

The General Council and Register of Osteopaths had Diana, Princess of Wales as its President. In 1992 they held a Reception to which representatives of all the affiliated osteopathic organizations were invited, in order to meet the Princess. I knew that she had experienced treatment and it was good to hear her speak with such enthusiasm about it.

In 1992 I renewed contact with John Wernham. Given that both our schools needed to move to larger premises it seemed worthwhile to explore at least the possibility of our two organizations getting together again. There were obvious advantages in pooling resources if, and it was a big *if*, the osteopathic differences of the past could be resolved. We agreed to keep in touch. Our confidential meetings continued, in fact we even viewed some properties together.

Returning to our search for validating authorities, none of the universities with which we had discussions had proved suitable for our particular needs. Then Paula Fletcher wrote to the University of Wales, the largest external degree validating body in the U.K. The response was encouraging. I remember so clearly the day the four of us visited Cardiff. The university representatives could not have been more helpful and positive. The distance separating our two organizations was not ideal but, apart from that, everything else was exactly what we had been looking for and without hesitation we decided in favour of Wales. Throughout they were efficient, supportive and it was a delight to work with them. In 1993 the University of Wales validated our BSc (Osteopathy) General Degree with Honours. Subsequently, this was upgraded to a fully classified honours degree.

Dr Dudley Tee agreed to become Research Adviser to the E.S.O. in January 1993. At the time he was Clinical Director at King's College Hospital; he was also a Founder Trustee of the Research Council for Complementary Medicine. Dudley was no stranger to the school, in fact I well remember his first lecture which was when the school was in Paris as E.F.O. He spoke about the research he was doing with Parnell Bradbury on the role of the chemical mediator in spinal manipulation.

For many osteopathic reasons 1993 was a vintage year. On 1st of July the Osteopaths Bill received the Royal Assent and became the Osteopaths Act 1993. It reached the Statute Book with the support of the government, all the main political parties and the medical profession. Quite an achievement! E.S.O. graduate Simon Fielding had been the architect of the Bill, and the school expressed its gratitude for all his work over 10 years with the presentation of an inscribed silver paperweight bearing the emblem of the school. This took place on 24th July 1993 at a surprise party in his honour, held at the school. Osteopathy was the first complementary medical profession to achieve statutory self-regulation thereby laying down high standards of training and ethical conduct. For the general public regulation by statute provides the same safeguards as when a doctor or dentist is consulted.

At the same time as working on our BSc, we had also been developing our Masters programme with the University of Greenwich. From the outset Joyce Vetterlein had been very enthusiastic to get this underway and had spearheaded much of the activity. It was a modular programme over three years of part-time study, open to all osteopaths with a minimum of one year's full time clinical practice. Joyce was appointed Pathway Leader for the school. We worked with Professor Edwin Metcalfe who was Head of the School of Biological and Chemical Sciences at the University.

In May 1994 our Master of Science degree in Osteopathy, which was the profession's *first*, was validated by the University of Greenwich. On 28th June 1994 we held a reception to mark the inauguration of our academic partnership with the University. The formal agreement was signed by Dr David Fussey, Vice Chancellor of the University of Greenwich and myself as Principal of the school. The guest list included the Mayor and Mayoress of Maidstone, Mr Andy Smith from the Department of Health, several M.P.s and of course many representatives of the University and the osteopathic profession. The event was widely covered by the press.

The University had warned us that we may get only some 10 MSc students in the 1st year, perhaps building up to around 20 in the 2nd year. However, in the first half of the 1st year we had offered 43 places of which 32 were confirmed acceptances. It must have been timely.

Life never stands still and by the end of 1993 there had been several changes in faculty. Simon Fielding's increased workload for the profession was such that he could not fulfil his duties for the school and then, rather unexpectedly, my other vice principal announced that he too was moving on. Dr Nic Rowley had been a great asset and had made a considerable contribution to our preparation for degree status. His Danish wife, Kirsten, who was a medical herbalist, had become involved as well: she dealt with the design, layout and production of the degree documentation – which, incidentally, was highly praised by the University. On the personal level I valued their friendship as well but they were not to be dissuaded. They sold up everything and moved abroad.

The trustees agreed that the time had come for the school to have a full-time osteopathic vice principal. There was a good response to the advertisement but the selection committee agreed that one applicant stood out from the rest. Renzo Molinari was appointed vice principal and took up his full-time post in January 1994.

Designated status was confirmed in May 1994 which meant that students on the degree course would receive mandatory awards. Being private sector education the award, unfortunately, was only some 18% of the tuition fees plus a means-tested maintenance grant.

The search for premises continued relentlessly. At last one appeared that seemed worth pursuing – Mote House. After several visits I concluded that if the right kind of lease could be negotiated, and if the large amount of work that would need to be done proved to be within our financial capability, then Mote House could be the answer to our property quest. I arranged for the board and architect Ric Wilkinson to visit the site. Many opinions were expressed; finally it was agreed that we should investigate the feasibility of Mote House.

Meantime there were further discussions with the Maidstone College of Osteopathy. I was no longer talking solely to John Wernham, we had now broadened our debates to include our vice principals. After several cordial meetings we agreed to experiment for a year by incorporating three of their lecturers into our G.O.T. team for the teaching of classical osteopathy, or total body adjustment as it was now called. It was felt that this would give everyone the opportunity of cooperating in a practical way to see if it would work. The arrangement was to start at the beginning of academic session 1994–95.

In the meantime there were developments in all directions. The board asked me to write an outline business plan for the move to larger premises. Much of my time was being spent in pursuing Mote House whilst at the same time looking at other properties.

Soon after starting as vice principal, Renzo Molinari made contact with Maidstone Hospital which resulted in students having the opportunity to observe in the maternity unit, as well as being able to watch orthopaedic surgery.

Following our achievement of degree status, our colleagues of the Collège International d'Ostéopathie in St. Etienne expressed interest in starting a full-time degree course. We began discussions with the University of Wales. Finally, representatives made a two-day visit to C.I.D.O. at the end of which the University gave its approval.

The final outcome in 1995, was that years 1 and 2 were franchised to C.I.D.O. and would take place in St. Etienne. Years 3 and 4, the predominantly clinical years, would take place at the E.S.O. thus circumnavigating the problem of having an osteopathic clinic in France which, at the time, would have been illegal. This was a natural progression of the already well established working relationship with C.I.D.O. – and another first for the E.S.O. In addition it was hoped that this development would be of assistance to our French colleagues in their struggle for recognition.

I was in for a bit of a shock at a meeting regarding Mote House in the late autumn of 1994. It turned out that there was another osteopathic charity negotiating for the property. Unbelievably it was the Maidstone College of Osteopathy! I decided that this had to be the end of the road for any hopes of osteopathic unity in Maidstone and I wrote an appropriate letter to John Wernham. At the same time I advised his three lecturers that it was no longer possible for them to teach at the E.S.O. End of story! It was also the end of pursuing Mote House as the board decided against it.

Disappointment, it is said, should always be taken as a stimulant, and never as a discouragement. What next, I asked myself. I decided to write to some 25 estate agents, this time spelling out exactly what I was looking for. My vision had always been for a university campus environment – a large character property with plenty of land for future development and as near as possible to Maidstone.

Actually, ever since the 1970s I had been searching for properties for one reason or another. Sufficient space was an ongoing problem for the school. It seemed to grow quicker than we were able to provide the bricks and mortar. I suppose we had become a victim of our own success.

Only one estate agent out of the 25 replied. He rang me to say that I had described exactly a property that he had handled over a year ago but the sale fell through and it had been withdrawn from the market. I asked if he still had the details on file. He said he would put them in the post straight away and I might just get them before Christmas. I did – it was Boxley House Hotel.

Immediately following family festivities, Robert and I decided to go to the hotel for lunch. I recall that it was a bright, sunny but frosty morning. As we drove in, the sun was shimmering on the remaining frost which made the grass look as if it had been sprinkled with diamonds. The grounds were beautiful. As I got out of the car I said to Robert 'this is it, I know it'. (DADIRRI again perhaps) I was not bothered that it was not on the market. I felt sure I could get round that, as well as all the other problems that no doubt would present themselves. I know it sounds a bit 'Tinkerbellish' but if one believes in something enough, with a bit of luck and a tail wind chances are it will happen!

The board viewed the property after I had met the owners and ascertained that they would consider selling on condition that the negotiations were kept strictly confidential. Their previous abortive attempt at selling had greatly damaged their business so it was important to respect their wishes – but it was difficult to keep the identity of the property secret for such a long time. The board was in favour and everything was set in motion. From when I first heard about Boxley House until I was handed the keys it was 21 months – of hard work, neverending problems, and more ups and downs than a rollercoaster ride. It was necessary to remain focused, determined and optimistic but it was a trial of endurance to keep it all together *and* confidential. This was the culmination of a five-year search but

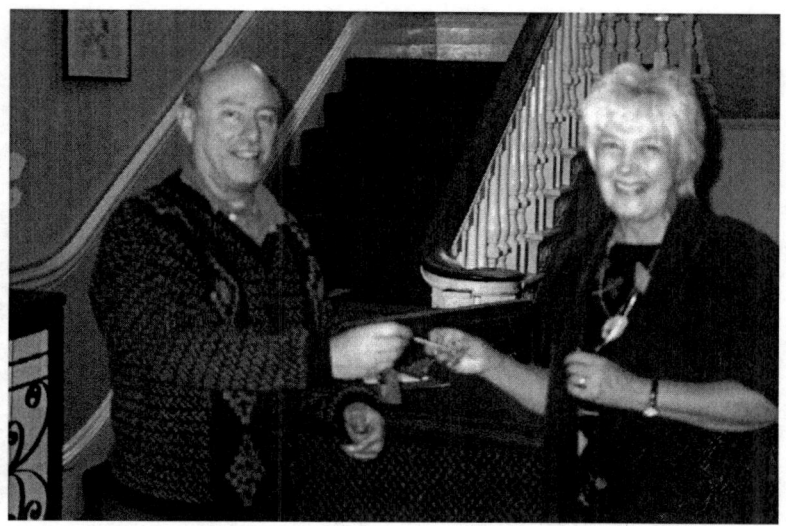

30th September 1996 – Margery receives the keys to Boxley House from Mr Fox

everyone who saw it subsequently agreed that Boxley House had been worth waiting for – students and staff were delighted with the school's new headquarters. It was appropriate that the keys were finally ours on the first day of the new academic session, 30th September 1996. This was an uncork the champagne moment!

There were some essential works to be carried out before we could move any classes to Boxley, and these were started straight away. The first and second years moved in at the beginning of the second term. Before then however we had our first event at the new premises. The University of Wales agreed that the degree programme (validated in 1993) would include the students who were in the second year at the time of validation as they had already been following the new curriculum. The first graduates therefore were in 1996 and to their great credit there was a 100% pass rate. Being a fairly rare result it brought pride

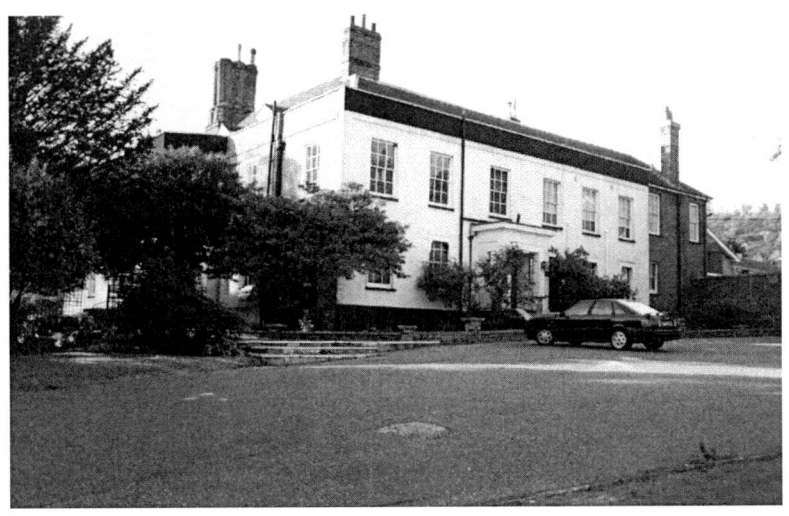

Boxley House dating from the early 17th century

and joy to all concerned. The presentation ceremony, attended by representatives of the University, was held in Boxley Church on 30th November 1996, followed by a reception and buffet

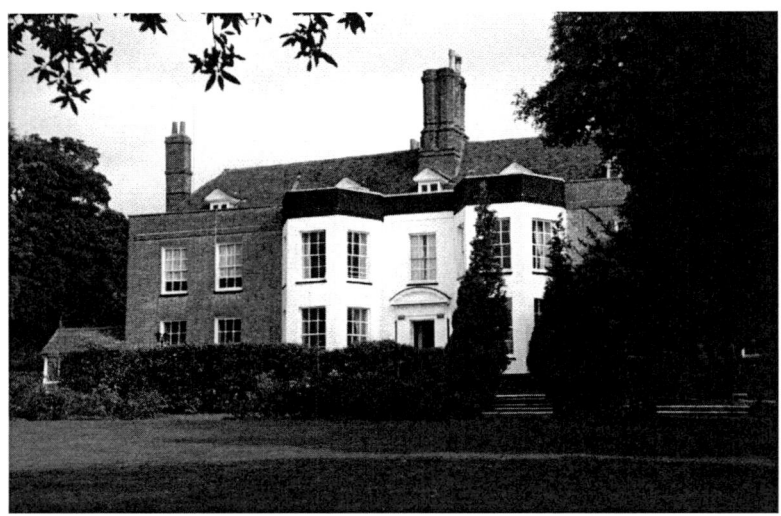

Boxley House with its south facing terrace

lunch at Boxley House. Just a week later we had a housewarming Christmas party for all the staff and what a happy occasion it was.

It seems like a small thing but it was really important to our graduates and colleagues across the Channel that our new address still had Maidstone in it. For them E.S.O. osteopathy and Maidstone were synonymous, so for the E.S.O.'s high profile abroad it mattered.

In January 1996 I received a telephone call from Dr Eric Thévenet with whom we had established a friendship over a number of years of his visits to Maidstone to lecture. We had lost touch for a while so it was great to hear that he was ringing me from London and yes, I was free for lunch and would get Robert to join us. Eric said he was with a friend (later to become his wife) and he wanted us to meet. It was Paloma Picasso. They were about to relocate to London so this was the first of many get-togethers.

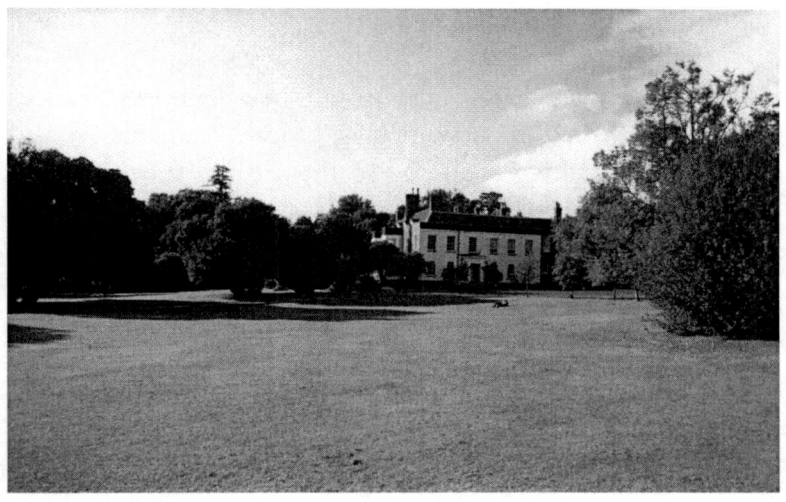

Boxley House is set in 17 acres of parkland

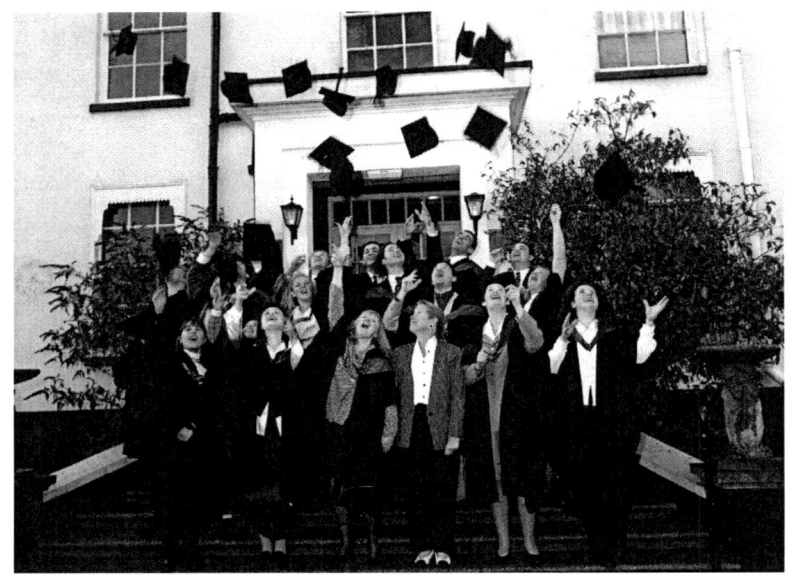

100% success rate for the first cohort of BSc graduates, 1996

Eric was very attached to the school. From his first visit with the Bobigny doctors he had watched it grow and was full of enthusiasm for its achievements.

When at last I had the keys to our new premises, we took Paloma and Eric to view Boxley House. Immediately they could see the potential and loved the setting. They offered to help us with our fundraising activities and in 1997 accepted to become patrons of the charity. Knowing how busy their lives were, it was a welcome boost personally to have the support of these dear friends and, from the school's perspective, their willingness to lend their names to our fundraising endeavours was greatly appreciated.

The link with Russia had been progressing well and Renzo had set up the course in St. Petersburg with E.S.O. lecturers making regular visits. By July 1997 it was time for us to receive the first group of Russian students in Boxley for a two-week seminar. We wanted to give them a special welcome and so we organised a reception attended by representatives from the Russian Embassy, the Mayor of Maidstone and other invited guests. On another occasion we entertained them at our home. A party with Russian friends is such a joyous experience. In no time they had made up a song about us and were all in full voice. They are always so appreciative and grateful.

Another memorable 1997 event was on the 2nd May when Robert and I were invited to John Wernham's 90th birthday celebration. It was a gathering of about 50 friends and family for a dinner in the Gate Tower at Leeds Castle. He gave a remarkable speech – but then he was a remarkable man.

On the 2nd December 1997 Renzo and I attended the University of Greenwich awards ceremony at Barbican Hall.

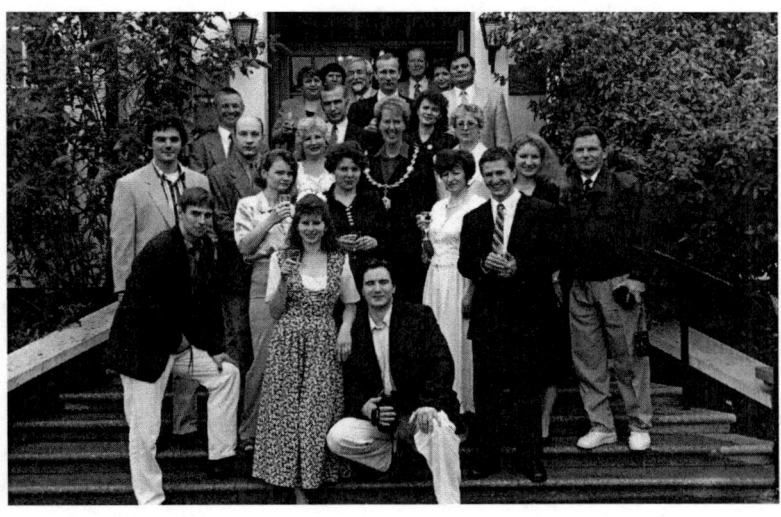

Our first group of Russian students in Boxley for a two week seminar

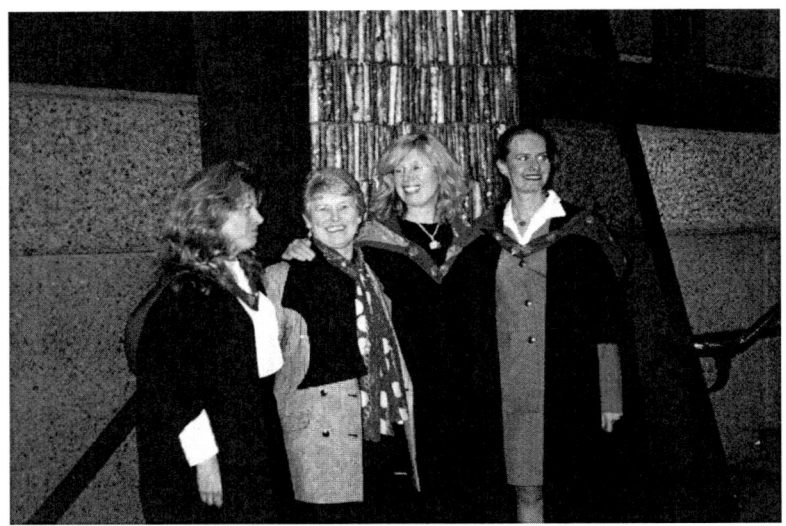

The first graduates of the first MSc Osteopathy with Margaret Jones, postgraduate coordinator

Our first three MSc graduates were Chris Conroy, Christina Szelinsky and Joyce Vetterlein – in fact these were the first ever MSc osteopathy graduates. It was a proud moment.

I had given a year's notice of my intention to retire as principal at the end of September 1997. There may have been one or two who would have preferred an earlier departure but I was determined to help the school achieve *all* the goals I had set for it at the beginning of my principalship – and we did just that. My only regret was that with all my other duties I did not have enough time to devote to fundraising. Even so, by 31.08.96 we had £325,189 in our designated development fund, the result of both fundraising and 'good housekeeping'. It was a useful sum towards our move to Boxley, but a lot more was needed to push things forward. We had the plans and the planning permission for a clinic and classroom development – all that was needed was the money!

After much discussion with the board, finally agreement was reached. I offered a year of full-time fundraising, without remuneration, in the hope that this would kick-start the process thus allowing the development of the site at Boxley to begin. In addition, to keep au fait with the school's progress, I would continue as company secretary for as long as it proved useful.

The time was right for the E.S.O. to have an osteopath at the helm once again and the choice was obvious. With so much more to be done internationally it was appropriate to have a European as principal. Renzo Molinari had been vice principal for three years, prior to that a lecturer and before that an E.E.O. student. It had been a long involvement and, above all else, I knew that he too loved the school.

The handover took place during the faculty weekend just prior to the new academic session 1997/98. Of course there was a big 'Farewell to Margery, Welcome to Renzo' party on the Saturday evening in true E.S.O. style. It was all very touching.

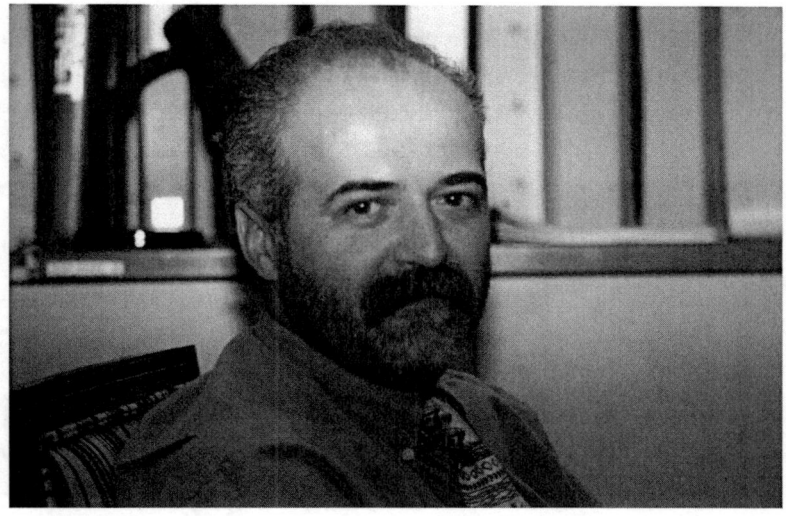

Renzo Molinari the new principal, 1st October 1997

I was satisfied that I was handing over an organisation that was sound on every level. The E.S.O. was recognised as one of the world's premier osteopathic educational institutions. We had the confidence of the universities with which we were involved, indeed Wales considered the E.S.O. as *the* osteopathic model at the centre of European development of the profession. Our first cohort of BSc degree students had attained 100% pass rate and our first MSc graduates were about to receive their awards. Our postgraduate and international departments were very active and our new green and beautiful premises had met with full approval. Financially our situation was sound and the five year projections I had done showed the way ahead for future development.

The board had decided to appoint a bursar to take over the financial and administrative aspects of my job, and Bob Read was chosen for the role. October until Christmas 1997 was to be the handover period during which I would have time to explain everything, tie up all the loose ends and clear my desk.

Towards the end of this period, I was working one day with Bob Read at Boxley when I received an urgent telephone call from my husband asking me to come home as he felt unwell – and he was. Various consultations and tests followed and within a couple of weeks he had surgery for cancer – but much worse was yet to come.

I was not able to start the fundraising until February and I decided to work from home so that I could look after Robert. There was a lot of preparatory work to be done – writing fundraising brochures, leaflets, posters, deeds of covenant and gift aid forms, the annual report etc. and in close consultation with Renzo of course, establishing a new house style to reflect the school's new green environment.

In 1998 Renzo was giving a lot of thought to a European academic osteopathic network and in July he arranged a conference with all the principals and representatives of the osteopathic schools and groups with which we were in touch. His ideas were received with enthusiasm, O.S.E.A.N. (Osteopathic European Academic Network) was born and an international conference was envisaged for the year 2000.

Renzo was invited by the University of Wales to sit on the validation panel when other osteopathic schools submit applications for degree status. A further honour came his way when he was nominated as European Representative of the American Academy of Osteopathy.

During the last year or so of my principalship I had wanted the E.S.O. to develop community-based projects. We had wrestled with the difficulties of trying to set up a drop-in clinic for those who could not afford even our modest fees. Although we were all agreed that it would be beneficial for the students to experience working with the severely disabled and disadvantaged members of the community, we had not found a way forward. Then, just after I had retired, I read an article in the local press about the community centre which sounded as if it could provide exactly what was needed. I passed it over to Renzo and, some months later, the school opened an osteopathic drop-in clinic in the Maidstone Community Support Centre in Marsham Street.

The launch on 7th October 1998 was heralded with town crier and mayoral attendance, and was tied in with National Back Pain Week, at the end of which we held a 'Focus on Boxley' weekend. This latter event was not so much a fundraiser as a PR exercise to make local people aware of the school and its work. The family event opened with majorettes, a marching

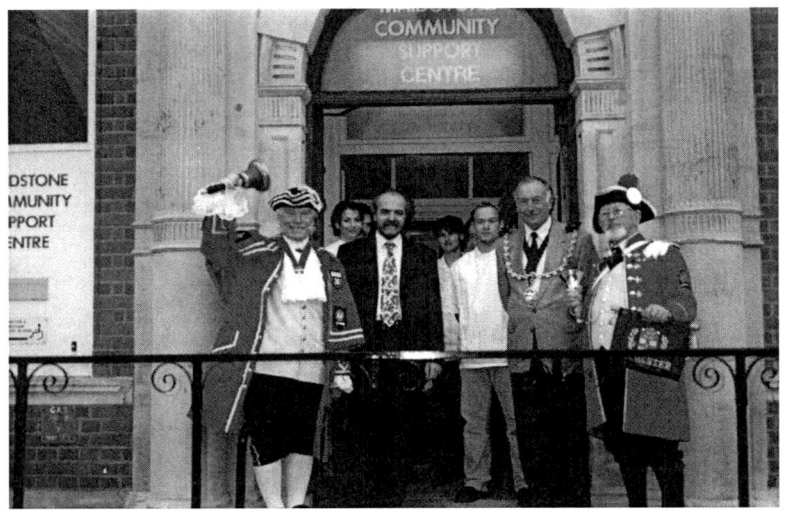

The launch of the osteopathic drop-in clinic in the Maidstone Community Support Centre

band and the release of hundreds of balloons. There were Morris dancers, Kentish music and specialist dancing groups, children's entertainment including clowns, stilt walkers,

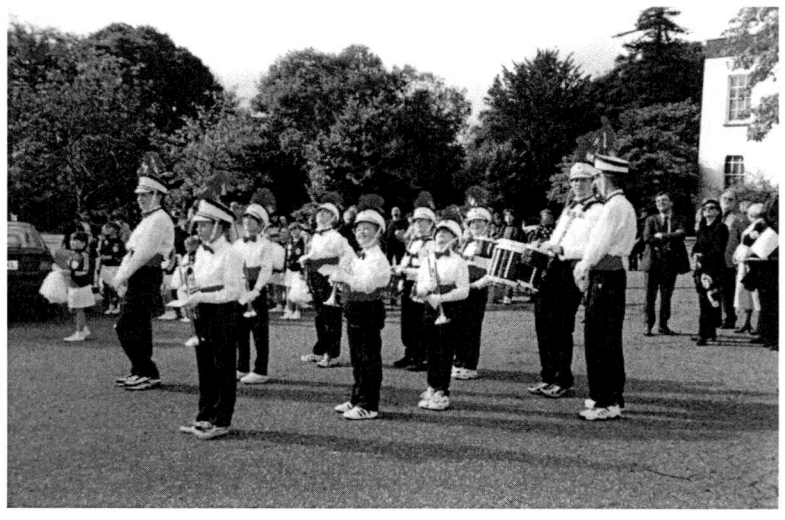

Focus on Boxley opened with marching band

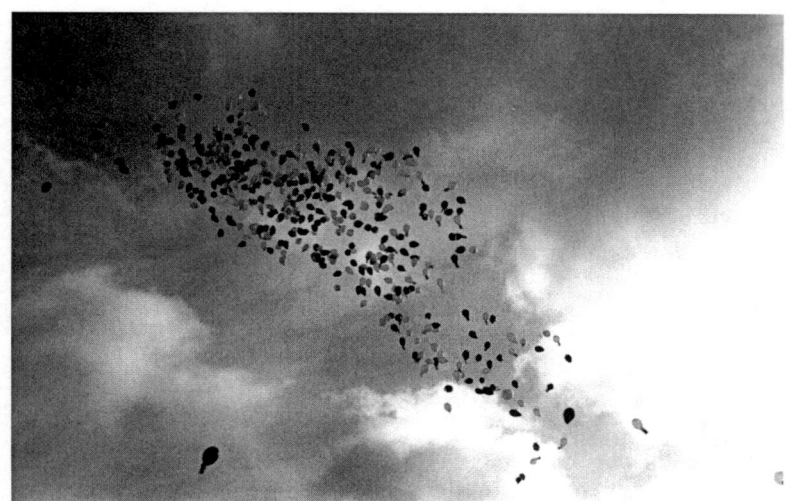

Focus on Boxley and the release of hundreds of balloons

juggling, balloon modelling, face painting, stalls with displays and tastings of Kentish foods, craft exhibits – and of course, talks on osteopathy and the school. The local church and the King's Arms pub joined in 'Focus on Boxley' with their own events. Our patrons Paloma Picasso and Eric Thévenet kindly attended and met local personalities over a Kentish luncheon. If nothing else, we had certainly introduced the E.S.O. to the village of Boxley. Following the event, it was interesting how many local people told me they had decided to make an appointment at the clinic.

In November of 1998 the school took the decision to keep the clinic at 104 Tonbridge Road for the next five years and carry out refurbishment. This of course removed the focus of the fundraising plans I had developed, but I knew it would not be my problem for much longer. There was no way I could complete the year I had offered, as my husband's health was deteriorating rapidly. At long last vascular dementia had been diagnosed, surely the cruellest of all diseases. It is the gradual disintegration both mentally and physically, that is so heartbreaking. I nursed him for seven years.

At the E.S.O., Renzo and his team were hard at work preparing for the inspection by the statutory body, the General Osteopathic Council, which was part of the process of accreditation of osteopathic schools.

It was a busy year as a full review of the MSc programme, and a quality assessment audit were also in progress. The outcome was successful revalidation by the University of Greenwich of the masters programme.

Good news academically came from the D'Oyly Carte Charitable Trust by way of research funding of £21,000 over three years to support a PhD programme. Considerable interest was shown and in the fullness of time it was to be another first for the E.S.O. – a PhD in osteopathy.

The universities and colleges admission service (U.C.A.S.) had accepted the membership application from the school, with effect for students entering in September 1999.

At the graduation ceremony in July 1999 I was presented with the E.S.O. Medal of Honour, as was Peter Blagrave and Stephen Pirie. Since then quite a number of other faculty members have received the medal. Peter and Stephen were delighted, and I knew I *should* have been but I wasn't. If the school wanted to acknowledge long and loyal service – great, but if the idea was to honour the co-founders then there should have been a posthumous one for Tom as well which could have been presented to his widow. Also I think it would have been preferable to have been a totally different medal – or some other symbol. Well, there, I have voiced my opinion and sincerely hope it does not upset anyone. At least I did not do a 'Beatles' and send it back! In the big scheme of things it is totally unimportant anyway. The school and its progress are what really count and the year 2000 was full of important happenings.

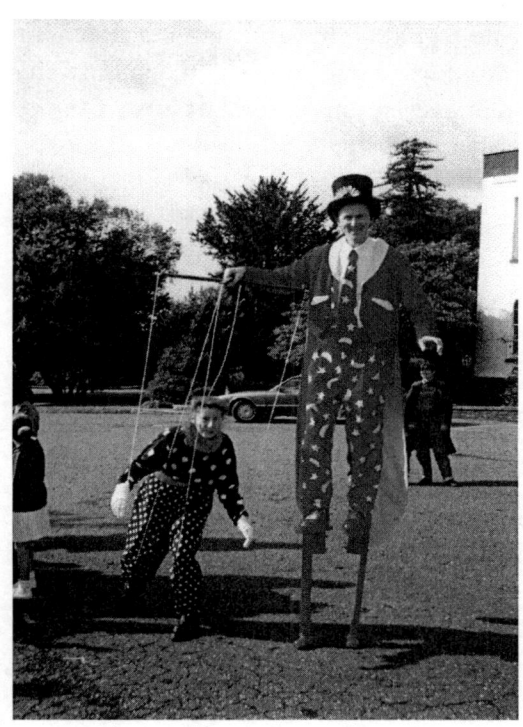

Focus on Boxley – plenty of entertainment for children.

There were two milestones. In May official notification was received that the Privy Council had approved the General Osteopathic Council's recommendation that the E.S.O. be an accredited institution for the training of osteopaths. This success was fundamental to the future existence of the school and worthy of a celebration as is E.S.O. custom.

The other event of huge significance was O.S.E.A.N.'s excellent international conference. When I first saw Boxley House I remember thinking what a wonderful venue it would make for a big international conference. Now at last it was taking place – on the 7th, 8th and 9th July 2000 with more than 250 delegates attending from over 20 countries. There were three days of lectures, practical workshops and demonstrations plus plenty of time for debate regarding research and developments in Europe. The whole event was inspirational and demonstrated the E.S.O.'s leadership in Europe and beyond. It was a triumph for Renzo and his team, in particular Corinne who did most of the organising.

The Council of Validating Universities approved the E.S.O. as an associate member in June.

Another year 2000 event was the appointment of a fundraising consultant, and a fundraising and development sub-committee was created.

The board asked me if I would accept to become a patron of the school. I was pleased to take on this new role and, as required by the board, resigned as company secretary.

2001 saw the structuring of O.S.E.A.N. Renzo as ever was doing a lot of travelling. In his ambassadorial function he was placing the school at the forefront of developments internationally, which was fulfilling all those aspirations we had from the very beginning of the school.

This is where my 50 years' history ends.

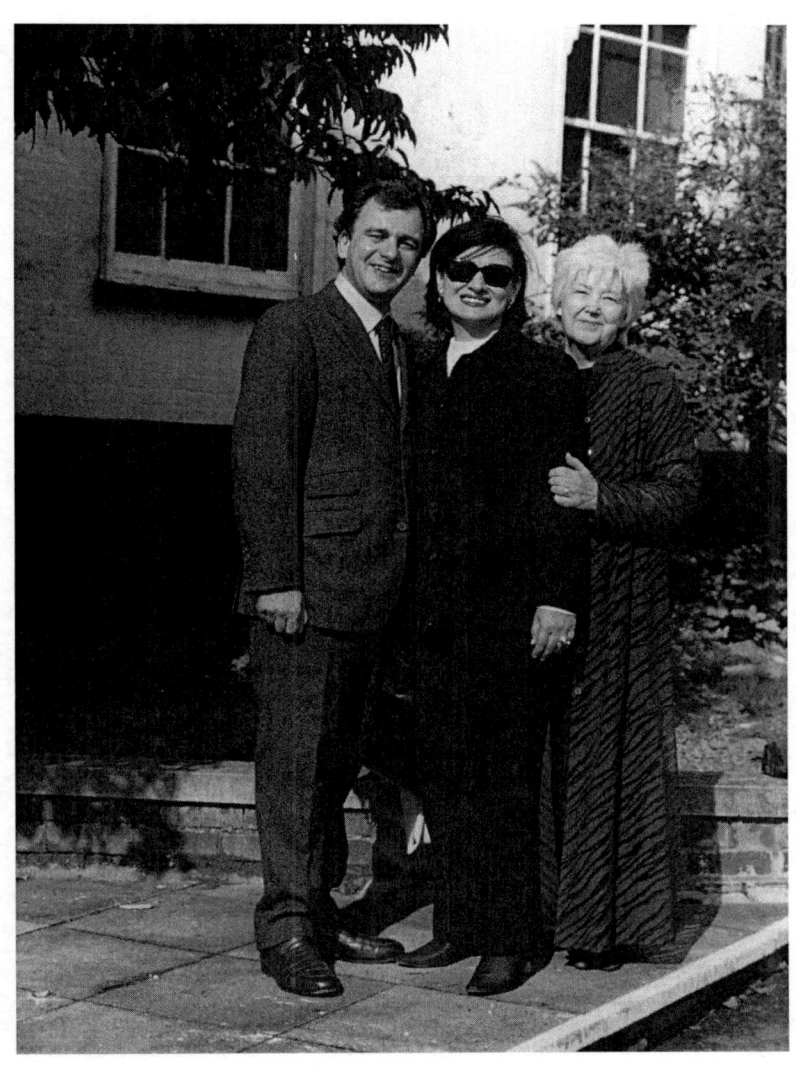

The three patrons of the school
Dr Eric Thévenet, Paloma Picasso Thévenet and Margery Bloomfield

Chapter Twelve

Unforgettable Osteopaths and some Unsung Heroes

'To teach is to learn' – Japanese proverb

THIS CHAPTER COULD run easily to the length of *War and Peace*. To avoid that happening I am going to confine my reminiscences to those osteopaths with whom I had a strong connection and who are no longer with us.

In the early days there were so many 'characters' in the profession both here and abroad. This was probably something to do with the pioneering spirit and all the battles that had to be fought on so many fronts, in the interests of osteopathic progress.

The following is a collection of memories – some running to several pages, others just snatches of moments in time. Above all I am deeply grateful that I had the good fortune to know them.

Tom Dummer was a part of my life for a very long time and I guess I knew him better than most. To recap we met in 1959, married seven weeks later, separated 1974, divorced 1979 – and both remarried within the same year. Whatever the ups and downs we never stopped working together. Even after Tom retired as principal we were still in constant touch so by the time of his death in May 1998 we had been working together for just on 40 years. For quite a few of those years it was difficult, but our focus was the school and that mattered above all else.

Although I have written quite a lot about Tom in this book (how could I do otherwise in writing the history of the school!), nevertheless there are some gaps that need filling.

Tom was a remarkable practitioner, a true master of osteopathy. He brought his creative side as a musician to the art of osteopathy, taking it to another dimension. Gez Lamb once wrote 'to see him at work was an education in the "inner game" of our remarkable discipline'. His open mind brought a breadth of vision to the teaching in the school. Was he a good lecturer? Well, he was sometimes the butt of students' sketches in our Christmas Revues, because his rather monotone voice could put some of them to sleep. That to one side, Tom's teaching and his enthusiasm for his subject inspired students.

He had a deep interest in all branches of natural therapeutics and practised several of them with great skill but, as time went on, he gradually dropped them in favour of his passion for osteopathy which ultimately dominated his professional life. He was involved too in the politics of the profession nationally and internationally and spearheaded much of its development.

I have seen in print that Tom was a life-long Buddhist. This is not correct. When I first met Tom he was 44 and knew nothing of Buddhism. As a matter of fact I was the one who had books on the subject having been given a copy for my 26th birthday of the Hermann Hesse novel *Siddhartha*. It was one of those life changing reads and my interest in Buddhism and attraction to all things Eastern has never left me. It was on our travels in India in the late 1960s when we visited the important Buddhist sites that our interest was kindled. On return home we joined the Buddhist Society but in 1974 when we separated I let my membership lapse because it just felt inappropriate to continue on the same philosophical path together when in reality we were going off in different directions. In that same year Tom formally took refuge with the Ven. Lama Chime Rinpoche and his studies in Buddhism continued and deepened. He also studied Tibetan medicine and wrote a book under that title in 1988. The two main osteopathic books he wrote were *Specific Adjusting Technique* in 1995 and *Textbook of Osteopathy* in two volumes which he completed just before his death in 1998.

On 2nd and 3rd June 2001 we had a Tom Dummer weekend of lectures and memories including the dedication of the Tom Dummer memorial bench in the garden to the left of the front door of Boxley House. The beautiful stone bench was designed and built by the caretaker Ares Perdios. I remember in the speech I made that day I put my order in for one exactly the same, when it's my turn to step off the bus.

On the Saturday evening we had a dinner dance which was followed by a fundraising auction. There were several lots but the star item was something that I was able to donate. It was the original typed manuscript of Fryette in a red leather binding, which had belonged to Teddy Hall. On Hall's death John Wernham gave all his memorabilia to the school but the Fryette he made me promise to keep personally, to avoid the risk of it disappearing from the library. This seemed like the moment to let it help the school's fundraising. There was a great deal of interest and the bidding was really exciting. Barrie Savory had pushed it up to £5,250. Finally it was his, but with typical generosity he paid up and then presented it back to the school. A great note on which to end the evening.

In view of the above this is an apt moment to recount some memories of **T. Edward Hall**. To some he was 'Tommy' but we always called him 'Teddy', although I am told he actually preferred 'Edward'. We often used to dine with him and I always looked forward to it as he was such a colourful character, full of stories, enthusiasm and humour. To watch him work was mind-blowing – what extraordinary ability he had. He lived for osteopathy. We were indeed fortunate to have him as Professor Emeritus of the school.

After a long illness Teddy Hall died on the 24th March 1979. We were grateful to be the recipients of his books and osteopathic memorabilia and named our library after him. I recall that I had his bookcase-desk in my office for many years, finally handing it over to Renzo Molinari when he took over from me as principal. His drawings by Stephen Ward still hang on the wall at the school, and I treasured as well his Boneshakers Club silver platter with all its signatures, as well as his diploma signed by J.M. Littlejohn.

In the early days **Paul Gény** was not just a colleague or friend, he was more like a member of the family. Between our monthly visits to Paris prior to 1965, and his monthly stays with us when he was working in the practice, plus some holiday time at their house in Brittany, we did spend quite a lot of time together. As the school developed, and then moved to Maidstone, we saw less and less of him. We always tried to persuade him to attend our various landmark celebrations but mostly without success.

There is something I have seen in print which needs correcting. The E.F.O. (Paris) was *not* shut down by the police and Paul did *not* go to gaol (see chapter 2 for the facts).

It is strange the funny little memories that linger. One Christmas I made up a hamper for Paul to take home to Paris with all the usual English festive goodies e.g. smoked salmon, stilton and walnuts, port, Scottish shortbread etc, plus of course brandy butter and a luxury Christmas pudding. I gave Paul strict instructions about how to deal with the pudding. When we saw him again early in the new year it turned out that everything was delicious *except* for the pudding: the instructions got lost in translation and the pudding was emptied out of the basin into a saucepan of hot water which was then simmered for two hours. Imagine!

I first met **Ange Castejon** in January 1960 whilst on my honeymoon with Tom in Paris (as previously related, at one of the E.F.O. seminars).

Ange qualified as a physiotherapist in 1948, which was also the year he married Geneviève. Later he studied with Dr Jarricot and it was at one of Jarricot's seminars that he met Paul Gény, in 1953. This was a meeting that changed the direction of his life. Later he joined the Ecole Française d'Ostéopathie in Paris, obtaining his D.O. in 1960. From that moment, having closed his physiotherapy practice, Ange was an osteopath and indeed one of the pioneers of osteopathy in France. He played a pivotal role firstly in the development of the E.F.O., giving great support to Paul Gény, and again when the school moved to England he was involved at every step with the progress of the Ecole Européenne d'Ostéopathie. In spite of innumerable fines for the illegal practice of medicine, Ange continued resolutely to treat and to teach osteopathy. He and Geneviève had two sons, one of whom, Christian, followed in his father's footsteps, obtaining his D.O. from the E.E.O.

Ange and Geneviève were dear friends over a very long time. They were renowned for their warm and generous hospitality.

There is a story I must tell – against myself – but Peter Blagrave will never forgive me if I omit it. A seminar coupled with an E.E.O. meeting in Lyon had been arranged and a few of us had been invited to dinner at the Castejons on the evening before it was due to begin. Robert and I arrived about 7.30pm along with Maurice Sainte-Rose. Tom and Jo were on their way but delayed... and delayed... so whilst waiting we were offered delicious champagne cocktails – again and again... We finally had dinner about 11pm and when we left the Castejon apartment we were all verging on the legless. Back at our hotel I knew that Peter Blagrave would have arrived so I walked up and down the street outside the hotel singing out his name. He has never let me forget that!

Parnell Bradbury, P.B., as we always called him, was a man of many parts: osteopath, researcher, prolific writer, author, playwright and actor. He and Tom were close friends and worked together for many years. Tom used to see patients in P.B.'s Sussex practice once a week on a Friday. I used to join them in the evening and we would go out to dinner. P.B. was great company, flirtatious, impish even, but always interesting. He was a graduate of the B.S.O. but was ever fascinated by 'the hole in one' of B.J. Palmer.

P.B.'s books included *Healing by Hand, Adventures in Healing* and *The Mechanics of Healing (Spinology)*. In the 1960s in association with Dr Dudley Tee, P.B. established that specific high velocity adjusting of notably the upper cervical and mid-dorsal areas in many instances did facilitate the release of a chemical mediator.

P.B. worked over many years on his Specific Adjusting Technique (S.A.T.) in accord he said with Still's principle of 'Find it, fix it and leave it alone'. During all this period Tom had been working with him on the positional lesion and when P.B. died Tom went on refining this minimal treatment approach and making S.A.T. his own.

Last but by no means least of my Unforgettable Osteopaths is **John Wernham** or J.W. as he was often called. In these pages I have written a great deal about him already, but there are some more personal stories that I would like to relate.

John was a difficult man, at times very difficult, but he was also very special. I was ever mindful of the fact that without his help on more than one occasion the E.E.O./E.S.O. would never have survived. Of course we disagreed often and argued hotly many times but somehow our personal relationship survived, aloof from all the storms. When my Robert got to know John he too found a real connection with him. They would often exchange letters or telephone calls, rarely about osteopathy, but other interests they had in common like printing and publishing, and whenever J.W. brought out a new publication he would always send Robert a copy. We had a deep and abiding affection for John, which I think was reciprocated.

As I write now I am sitting in what used to be his chair and at what used to be his desk. He gave me these two items of furniture back in the 1970s and I have used them ever since.

When I was still married to Tom there was an occasion when he was invited to lecture, which involved him being away overnight. John and his wife Jess invited me to stay with them for the weekend. We went out to dinner at the old Royal Star Hotel on the Saturday evening and Sunday morning I was well and truly spoilt by Jess with breakfast in bed. The rest of the time we sat and talked. John showed me some of his amazing photographs. He had a career in photo-journalism before taking up osteopathy and, during the war, he was in the film and photographic section of Military Intelligence in Africa. It was such a relaxing and bonding couple of days, I have never forgotten it.

The Maidstone Osteopathic Clinic Committee asked me to arrange a 70th birthday celebration party for John at the clinic on the 2nd May 1977, which I was very happy to do. It was well attended and greatly enjoyed by colleagues, friends, lecturers and students. I know J.W. was touched by the warmth of everyone's good wishes and the presentations but he found it almost impossible to express thanks. The following day he came downstairs to my office and we had a cup of tea together and talked about nothing in particular. I knew that was his way of saying how much he appreciated his party.

We invited John to the school's 25th anniversary celebration (which was long after we had parted company with him) and we were delighted that he accepted. Robert waited at the front door for his arrival and then escorted him through to the lecture hall. Spontaneously everyone jumped to their feet and gave him a standing ovation, and I know he was both surprised and touched by the gesture. It was a memorable moment.

J.W. had always said that he intended to live until he was 90. In fact he outstripped even his own expectations. He was still riding his bicycle to the clinic well into his 80s. In a weird kind of way I expected him to live forever but death is not an optional extra. He went on treating patients until the end and died after a brief illness just short of his 100th birthday. I represented the school at his funeral.

...and some unsung heroes

In an osteopathic school praise and appreciation tend to centre on the osteopathic stars. Although this is understandable, I would like now to sing the praises of all those – past and present – who have contributed to the life of the school. Each and every one has had a part to play and, as we all know, 'the whole is only as good as the sum total of its parts.' Being something of a workaholic myself I tended to attract those similarly afflicted – which is probably why we achieved so much. Let us begin with academic advisers.

Ann Carroll came out of retirement to work with us and the school owes her a debt of gratitude for all she did to help us on our way. As our education consultant, she was not immediately popular with students and some staff because of her rather strict demeanour, but when people got to know her they realised how helpful she was, whatever the problem. I always appreciated Ann's wise counsel and I learned a lot from her. After she retired – again – she joined the board of trustees.

Following Ann, I was delighted to appoint **Dr Paula Fletcher** as our educationalist – and she is still with the school. Having been through various titles along the way, Paula is now vice principal (academic). If there were awards for hard workers, Paula could well snatch first prize! She has worked tirelessly for the school for the past 20 years, helping it over the various academic hurdles of BSc, MSc and PhD. I enjoyed working with Paula, due in large part to her dry humour and occasional profanity!

It was Ann Carroll who introduced us to **Peggy Head** who became a voluntary worker, doing all manner of useful jobs. She was a skilled flower arranger, dealt with the post, ran messages, helped out in the library and anywhere else she was needed – and always with a smile. Peggy really loved the school – and it was warmly reciprocated.

The French side of our operation was very fortunate with its interpreters. We had **Martine Faure-Alderson** first, about whom I wrote in chapter 3, then **Françoise Golden**. Over the years she took on added responsibilities and became an executive assistant and I remember how helpful and supportive she was during the E.E.O.'s 'troubled patch'. With equal good fortune we then found **Mira Shapur** who, until a couple of years ago, was still interpreting for the school – at her usual lightning speed.

Marilia Vasquet's appointment as directrice d'études francophones was a great success – and took a huge amount of work off my shoulders. The francophone students were delighted with her efficiency, tact and Gallic charm. Marilia, being multilingual, was a great asset given the growth of our international activities.

I must include in my unsung heroes' list **Len Austin**, our loyal taxi driver. It was Tom who 'found' Len, he used to drive him to and from school. Then we began to use Len for airport runs and today he is still providing that ever punctual and reliable service.

When we first moved into 104 Tonbridge Road we had difficulty finding good cleaners, then I met **Paul Fryer** who was about to start a cleaning business. I think we were his first big account.

His business grew rapidly and he began to include garden and ground maintenance. Nearly 30 years on Paul is still keeping everything clean and tidy.

We have had some long serving members of the board of O.E. & R. Ltd, as well. **Wadie Manston** was one of the first trustees and served as treasurer, never missing a meeting, until his death in 1997. **Phil Adams** was another early addition to the board who remained a member until her death. From the start of the full-time course and the incorporation of the company in 1974, **John Barkworth** has been involved with the school. He became a member of the board in 1988 and later its chairman. In the early days we always referred to the board members as governors, now we say the board of directors and trustees. Whatever we call them, they are hard working, unpaid and have a lot of responsibility.

We also have some very long-serving members of faculty. **Peter Blagrave** joined the faculty a year or so after the school's arrival in England, **Stephen Pirie** and **Robert Lever** both became involved with the start of the full-time course – and all three are lecturing still. Two others who are still there having joined following graduation are **Gez Lamb** in 1982 and **Anna Reeve** 1988. Then of course there is **Leslie Smith**, still teaching physiology and providing the summer science course. I wonder if Leslie remembers his first time at the school. I was entertaining a visiting French colleague to lunch in my office when Leslie arrived, a little early for his interview so I invited him to sit down at the table and join us. It was all a touch informal as interviews go – but he got the job. Leslie told me later that he decided there and then he would love to work in such a lively and unusual place!

There are so many more members of faculty I would like to mention, but I fear this book could well turn into a 'Directory' instead of a 'History' so I must stop.

With clinic numbers building up rapidly it became necessary to appoint a clinic administrator. In 1988 **Pearl Thurston** (later **Richards**) took on the task and managed with great efficiency to streamline the running of the clinic.

She was followed by **Elizabeth Gower** who brought additional abilities to the job being a capable first aider – and another very hard worker. Elizabeth was still in post when I retired.

Then there were all the clinic receptionists starting with **Enid**, then that wonderful double act **Stephanie and Tamara** who went on to administrative clinic jobs, and **Lynn** – and so many others. Tamara is still there. Support staff are hugely important to the smooth running of all schools, and we were fortunate in having a great admin team. It started of course just with me then, at last, we were able to afford a part-time secretary, **Jenny**. The first full-timer was **Catherine** who later needed an assistant **Debs** – and so the team kept on building. There was **Anne, Sue, Jacquie, Sylvie, Jo, Dee, Yvonne, Gill, Sheila, Cathy** – and **Corinne** who, like Jacquie, is still working at the E.S.O., both now having important administrative positions.

The librarians in my time were **Lesley Bryce**, then **Sarah O'Callaghan** followed by **Ray Smith** who was still in post when I retired.

Our first caretaker was **Sue Terry** who had fulfilled those duties originally for John Wernham. When we moved to 104 Tonbridge Road, Sue asked if she could move with us and so together with husband Gordon and cat, Sam, they were installed in the flat on the top floor.

Sue (Mrs T) became our caterer as well. With an increasing number of vegetarians in the school I recall sending Sue on a caterers Cordon Vert cookery course run by the Vegetarian Society. Everyone was delighted with the variety of dishes she produced as a result of her professional diploma. Soon Sue needed extra help in the kitchen and she was ably assisted by her friend **Irene**. Sue had a great sense of occasion and whenever there was something special going on (which was frequently!) she could always rise to the challenge.

When our move to Boxley House grew imminent Sue decided to retire and we gave her a warm farewell party in April 1997.

We interviewed many couples for the post of caretakers for our newly acquired Boxley premises. It was clear that **Gerald and Janet Buckfield** were an ideal choice as they brought a range of skills to their jobs. Gerry had been a builder and he did a lot of useful work on Boxley House. He could take on the role of 'butler' just as easily when the need arose. Janet was an experienced and efficient housekeeper and together, they brought warmth and support for the students as well.

Joanne Paterson was appointed caterer and together with her colleague **Fiona Gillard** produced some memorable food.

As Boxley House was previously a hotel, it had an On licence and an entertainment licence, and we decided to keep both. I became licensee together with the Buckfields, after we had attended the obligatory course and passed the National Licensees Certificate Examination. I remained licensee for some years after I retired – although I never did get around to pulling a pint!

We were sad to say farewell to Gerry and Janet when they accepted the offer of a job they could not refuse, and went off to live in France.

After I retired it was dear **Vivienne and Ares Perdios** who were appointed caretakers.

*

Before finishing my homage to all the unsung heroes, I would like to pay tribute to my late husband **Robert** who did so much for the school in so many ways and most of it nobody ever knew about.

If, as I have claimed, I married osteopathy and Tom, then it must follow that Robert married osteopathy and Margery.

In 1972 when Robert accepted the part-time post of liaison officer of the I.F.P.N.T. he also learnt from us about the school's activities and became very interested. Understanding how overworked we were, coupled with the tight financial situation, he immediately offered his services to the school as well – but free of charge – and this continued for a decade.

Eventually the situation was regularised by the board who gave Robert (or Bob as everyone else called him) the title of development consultant with a modest retainer; he also became an ex-officio member of the board.

He had many articles published about the school across a broad spectrum of journals. In 1976 to help the school's fundraising efforts, Robert produced (at his own expense) the cartoon booklet 'Oh, for an Osteopath' which raised around £1,500 and was very well received. A few years later he wrote/drew a sequel 'Oh for Another Osteopath' which raised another £1,000. He also started a newsletter for students – on a shoestring, largely a cut and paste job, typewritten and then photocopied. It was a fun publication, enjoyed by all.

There will be quite a few students who will remember Robert as a healer/counsellor/befriender. Anyone feeling the need for a chat – away from school premises – could call in anytime for a cup of tea.

If anyone asked me how I met Robert I used to reply 'My first husband advertised for him' – which was strictly true (see chapter 5) but needed amplification. Truth is often stranger than fiction.

Chapter Thirteen

...and in Conclusion

'Life can only be understood backwards but it must be lived forwards'

THE JOURNEY HAS come to an end, 1951–2001 – the first 50 years. For me personally it is also 50 years. I met Tom and heard about osteopathy for the first time in 1959 and I have written this book in 2009. What enormous changes I have seen.

It is for those who come after me to write about the next half century, but a word of advice if I may – do it in decade slices because chronicling 50 years in one go is a huge task. I feel as if I have just walked off the set of 'This Is Your Life'. In many ways it has been a strange experience regurgitating all this information which, inevitably, has encompassed a big chunk of my life. Powerful memories have been evoked – and not without some emotional moments.

Of course I have not covered *everything* – how could I – but I am confident I have included the major developments and happenings of the period. After all I did not set out to write the *Encyclopaedia Britannica* of osteopathy nor for that matter, the tell-it-all of the E.S.O. My aim was more modest: simply to record for posterity how it all began.

We may have started as a penniless cottage industry but we made progress at a phenomenal rate. To recap: 16 students started with the French school in exile, four years later we had a two-year waiting list. The full-time course started in 1974 with a small group of disgruntled students from elsewhere: eight years later the course was accredited by the G.C. & R.O. and within the next decade degree status had been achieved. I remember when I was writing the business plan for the purchase of Boxley House, I prepared a graph showing the school's progress since the incorporation of the sponsoring body O.E. & R. Ltd. Coopers and Lybrand who were overseeing the preparation of the business plan and doing the number crunching were highly complimentary about our 'impressive record'.

Looking back at how things were when I first became involved with osteopathy, one memory stands out: it was a man's world. Initially there were no women lecturing in the school and very few female students. Over the years the situation gradually changed until it reached the more or less stable 50/50 point. Of course high-flying business women were rare then as well.

In 1983 I was made a Fellow of the British Institute of Management and I decided I should attend some of their meetings. I recall one which was held at Leeds Castle. There were some 60 members present but I was the only woman. The other 'Fellows' did not seem to know what to do – make a fuss of me or ignore me completely. It was clear they decided on the latter. During the debate which followed the morning's lecture, I made some – apparently – useful suggestions and observations. Suddenly they began to take me seriously and during the lunch break I was quite overwhelmed with the attention!

When I became the first woman principal of an osteopathic school, I had a flashback to that awareness of being a woman in a man's world – but it soon passed. It was strange at first because I was doing essentially the same job I had always done but now I had a different title, which called for a change of mindset – and a slight shift in attitude. I told myself that an iron fist in a velvet glove was the best way forward.

In 1995, to my complete surprise, I was invited by Barclays Bank corporate manager to participate in the Kent Business Personality/Business Woman of the Year Awards. I did not win, but it was an interesting experience and good for the image of the school to have its principal nominated by the bank.

The school is not just about what is taught. It is also about the students and the staff, all those wonderful people who have made the E.S.O. We are all such a mix of strengths and weaknesses and every nuance in between. It is said that all organisations have their share of bad apples. I cannot recall any in the E.S.O. although, thinking about it, there were a few that were slightly bruised!

Personally I feel spoilt for riches with the people I have met and worked with on my osteopathic journey and I am full of admiration for every student who successfully graduates. It is a tough course calling for total commitment but the rewards are worth it. I doubt if there could be a more satisfying way to spend one's life than helping people.

Everyone used to say that the school was 'Margery's baby' and I suppose it was. Certainly I was there at the birth, and like all births, the pain was soon forgotten with the sheer joy of the new offspring. Teething problems soon followed and every now and again a bad attack of colic. The school's teen years were full of challenges – but that's puberty for you! With a lot of nurturing, the school finally came of age – degrees, achievements galore and all against the backdrop of statutory regulation. No wonder I felt like a proud mum!

There are a few questions which in various forms I have been asked repeatedly in recent years and I am going to attempt some answers. The first is a personal one: 'Margery, how did you come to live in Boxley?' In 1999 there was a whimsical story circulating in the school that I had liked Boxley so much I bought the village! I wish… Before moving we had a house in Bower Mount Road, just a couple of minutes from the school's Tonbridge Road premises, which was the sole reason we chose to live in Maidstone. I promised Robert that when I retired we would move.

Our long term plan was to relocate to France, travel a bit, take up painting, above all spend real time together doing lots of walking, reading and researching interesting topics to debate with friends over long, delicious dinners. The list of things we wanted to do in retirement was endless. Not one of them happened. 'Life is what happens when you are planning other things,' said John Lennon. It was true for him and it was true for us.

With the onset of Robert's illness, France was out of the question. Our next thought was the West Country but nothing came of that either. Then I asked Kentish Estate Agents to send us details of old character properties in small villages. Through the letterbox one day came details of The Old House, Boxley – absolutely the last village on earth that we would have considered, given that I was trying to remove myself from the E.S.O. However, someone I had met in the village told me it was a charming house and I should have a look. I did – and I fell in love with it. We made an absurd offer, which was refused, and so we put the idea of moving on the back burner. Robert's health – or lack of it – had to take precedence.

Many months later the estate agent rang to say the sale of The Old House had fallen through, the owners were taking it off the market unless by chance we were still interested and could improve on our first offer. The sum we would receive from the sale of our existing house was going to be the figure we would spend on any new purchase – and not a penny more, of that we were adamant.

The agent suggested putting our house on the market to ascertain what it would fetch. The first three couples to view all offered the full asking price but the last couple were not in a chain and wanted to buy there and then. We rang the owners of The Old House and made our best offer. They wanted £5,000 more. Stalemate. Then the following morning I received a cheque for £4,996 which I did not even know was owing to me! This sort of thing has happened to me a number of times in my life, and it's quite spooky. It feels as if everything is being orchestrated 'out there somewhere'. We decided not to fight it, £4 difference was not hard to find and so the deal was done. We moved in on New Year's Eve (of all nights) 1998/9. I have never regretted it. Boxley is a great place to live, with a terrific community spirit.

Knowing of my connection with the school, friends have posed the question 'what *is* osteopathy?' whilst osteopathic friends have asked if I have views on the future development of the profession, and, more recently, have asked if I have any specific hopes for the school or any advice to offer it.

Mindful of the fact that I am not an osteopath and, since retirement, much has changed which means I am no longer up to speed with the profession's progress, I question whether I should even venture an opinion. Be that as it may I am going to have a go.

In his excellent book *The Good Back Guide* published in 2006, Barrie Savory wrote in the front of the copy he kindly sent me: 'To Margery, the best osteopath never to have worn a white coat…' Clearly, Barrie's words have gone to my head and so I offer my thoughts – accept them or reject them – it matters not.

Perversely I am going to start with what osteopathy is *not*. It is *not* just techniques, it is *not* a kind of super-physiotherapy, it is *not* some kind of manipulative therapy, it is *not* an adjunct to orthopaedics, it is *not* just about treating back pain, even though it is best known for its successes in this area, but to limit it in this way is far removed from the principles laid down by the founder Dr. A.T. Still. Nor are patients a mere collection of bones to be adjusted into good health. There are several aspects to the human being and they must all be taken into account.

It was Still who coined the word 'osteopathy', which is a combination of two Greek words osteon (bones) and pathos (disease). It was perhaps an unfortunate choice as the layman might think the osteopath treats diseases of the bone, or that he is some kind of bone doctor – wrong in both cases.

So what is osteopathy?

It is not easy to say in a few words but if pushed to do so I would say probably – it is a philosophy, a science and an art. I realise that does not help very much. Over the years I have seen many definitions, but there is not an official one and I am sure that is a 'good thing'. Let me try again. It is a system of manual medicine with a distinct method of diagnosis based on Still's original precepts – structure governs function, and the rule of the artery is supreme. The second precept puzzled me when first I read it but then I discovered it was underlining the importance of a healthy blood supply and good drainage both venous and lymphatic.

Another of Still's fundamental principles was find it, fix it, and leave it alone – nature will do the rest.

The body produces its own medicines. Above all osteopathy is a philosophy of health care. It is a distinctive art and in its application it is vast. Intention is everything. Teddy Hall's words have remained with me always. 'Its spirit is creative with endless possibilities.'

I recall vividly that Simon Fielding spent an inordinate amount of time avoiding having a definition put into the Osteopaths Act. His argument that it could stifle the future development of the profession, eventually, was heard and understood by Ministers and so no definition was included. It would be a tragedy for the profession to impose such a definition on itself.

I have maintained always that the difference between a good osteopath and a brilliant one is Factor X. My guess is that Factor X is the presence and the touch of a healer. Of course osteopathy can be – and indeed is – taught to a very high standard but after graduating the interpretation and the application of osteopathic medicine is so individual.

Regarding the question about the profession, osteopathy now wears a mantle of 'respectability' since the advent of statutory regulation and degree status, but practitioners should remain vigilant. It is to be hoped that any regulations from 'on high' and/or university pressures do not put osteopathy in a straitjacket. Those who care deeply about preserving the identity of osteopathy must resist any attempt to whittle it down and reduce it to the lowest common denominator. Bullies come in all guises! Recently I have become aware of some disquieting trends. Let us hope they will be satisfactorily resolved. Osteopathy deserves its rightful place in health care.

The following are some generalisations plucked randomly from my experience of keeping the school on the straight and narrow financially, whilst guiding its expansion and development.

Big decisions have long term effects so it is really important to have a clear vision of the way ahead. As mentioned before, I am an advocate of three to five year plans. Too many changes of direction weaken an organisation. Big impressive plans are easy to make but there must be someone at the financial steering wheel who has full and complete knowledge of where the school is heading – and understand its heartbeat – in order to provide the long term projections and a business plan for the realisation of the project. In other words, someone must be able to connect the dots.

If heavy reliance on fundraising is in the equation then an enthusiastic, experienced person is a must to spearhead lots of ongoing activity.

Keeping the E.S.O. in the public eye is of paramount importance so that all its 'publics' are kept aware of the school – nationally, internationally and locally. During my time I was aware of the large number of osteopaths trained in other schools, who wanted E.S.O. graduates as assistants because they had 'an extra something' as one practitioner put it to me. If that ever ceased to be the case, it would be time to worry. The school must never lose its special flavour.

I recall something Renzo said to me when he was still a student. He told me he had chosen to study at the E.E.O./E.S.O.

because it had a heart and a soul, which in his view set it apart from other schools. Long may it be so.

Regarding hopes for the school, yes I have many. I hope some of the senior lecturers who have left can be persuaded to return in order to preserve the essential 'ESOness'. I hope the course will not become too medicalised. I hope the fundamental principles of osteopathy are always at the core of the curriculum. I hope the course will continue to be taught against a background of natural therapeutics. I hope the school will have always the ability to recognise when it has something important, whether animate or inanimate, and value it. I hope the school will never develop a tick box approach to administration.

I hope the E.S.O.'s leadership in the international field is maintained and enhanced further. I hope the intrinsic nature of the school is never lost, the essence that makes people say 'The E.S.O. is a special place.'

Finally, I hope the school will always be guided by the power of love, and never the love of power.

*

It is a constant source of joy to me that so many graduates, former staff and faculty keep in touch. As an added bonus, if they have a reason to go to Boxley House, they call in as well. *Please continue to do so.*

*

If you have been reading these pages, hopefully you have bought a copy of the history. Please encourage your friends and colleagues to do likewise because every pound from the sale of this book is going towards the creation of a bursary fund/lending scheme for E.S.O. students. I thought that would create an appropriate 'compost heap'!

In addition to writing the history, I am gathering together all my vast collection of photographs, press cuttings and memorabilia. I have earmarked scrapbooking as one of my next hobbies as I want to present them well for posterity. When the job is done I intend to give these gems of the past to the independent osteopathic archive which is being set up, and of which I have agreed to become a trustee.

My guess is that even those who have been around the E.S.O. for a long time may well have discovered some things in this history that they did not know. I am equally sure there will be some who will have a different perspective, whilst others may have a different memory of the same event.

There are certain books on osteopathy of which it is said that the real message is 'between the lines'. Perhaps this is one of them…

Above all I hope this history of the E.S.O. will evoke some happy memories – and give recent graduates and current students an idea of what it was like in the early days.

> *The Past is History*
> *The Future a Mystery*
> *The Present a Gift*
> *– which is why we call it* **the present**

Landmark Dates in the School's History

1951	School starts in Paris as Ecole Française d'Ostéopathie
1965	School moves to London
1971	The School is renamed Ecole Européenne d'Ostéopathie and moves to Maidstone, Kent
1974	Osteopathic Education and Research Ltd is incorporated as a limited liability company registered as a charity, and trading as European School of Osteopathy/ Ecole Européenne d'Ostéopathie
1974	The four year full-time diploma course starts
1978	The School buys 104 Tonbridge Road, Maidstone
1979	Following essential building works, the School moves in to 104 Tonbridge Road
1981	Relationship with Maidstone Osteopathic Clinic comes to an end
1982	School requests inspection by G.C. & R.O.
1983	Osteopathy's first custom built clinic built at 104 Tonbridge Road
1986	Decision taken to gradually run down the School's six year part-time 'Cours Francophone'
1987	Collège International d'Ostéopathie (C.I.D.O.) founded with full cooperation of the School
1989	School starts its Department of Postgraduate Studies
1993	University of Wales validates School's BSc (Osteopathy) General Degree with Honours
1994	Master of Science Degree in Osteopathy (the profession's first) validated by the University of Greenwich

Continued…

1995	Partial franchise of degree course to C.I.D.O.
1996	BSc programme upgraded to Full Honours
1996	School buys Boxley House
1998	First meeting of Osteopathic European Academic Network (O.S.E.A.N.)
1999	School launches PhD in Osteopathy programme
2000	School gains accreditation by the General Osteopathic Council
2001	School celebrates 50th Anniversary since inception in Paris

Abbreviations

A.O.A.	American Osteopathic Association
B.C.N.O.	British College of Naturopathy and Osteopathy
B.C.O.M.	British College of Osteopathic Medicine
B.N.A.	British Naturopathic Association
B.C.N.	British College of Naturopathy
B.N.O.A.	British Naturopathic and Osteopathic Association
B.O.A.	British Osteopathic Association
B.S.O.	British School of Osteopathy
C.B.O.	Collège Belge d'Ostéopathie
C.I.D.O.	Collège International d'Ostéopathie
C.O.F.	Collège Ostéopathique Français
D.H.	Deutsche Heilpraktikerschaft
E.E.O.	Ecole Européenne d'Ostéopathie
E.F.O.	Ecole Française d'Ostéopathie
E.S.O.	European School of Osteopathy
G.C. & R.O.	General Council and Register of Osteopaths (The Register)
G.Os.C.	General Osteopathic Council
G.O.T.	General Osteopathic Treatment
I.C.N.T.	International Committee for Natural Therapeutics
I.F.P.N.T.	International Federation of Practitioners of Natural Therapeutics

Continued...

I.L.E.A.	Inner London Education Authority
J.M.L.	John Martin Littlejohn
J.W.	John Wernham
M.C.O.	Maidstone College of Osteopathy
M.O.C.	Maidstone Osteopathic Clinic
M.P.	Member of Parliament
M.R.O.	Member of the Register of Osteopaths
O.C.C.	Osteopathic Centre for Children
O.E. & R. Ltd	Osteopathic Education and Research Ltd.
O.S.E.A.N.	Osteopathic European Academic Network
P.B.	Parnell Bradbury
P.P.C.N.T.	Paramedical Practitioners Committee for Natural Therapeutics
P.R.	Public Relations
S.A.T.	Specific Adjusting Technique
S.R.O.	Société de Recherchers Ostéopathiques
U.C.A.S.	Universities and Colleges Admission Service

REFERENCES

Every prospectus of the:

Ecole Française d'Ostéopathie (Londres)

Ecole Européenne d'Ostéopathie

European School of Osteopathy

Minutes of Board Meetings of Osteopathic Education and Research Ltd.

End of year Reports and Accounts of Osteopathic Education and Research Ltd.

E.S.O./E.E.O. Prinicpal's Reports

E.S.O. Newsletters

E.S.O./E.E.O. News Bulletins

E.S.O. News Bulletins

International Federation of Practitioners of Natural Therapeutics – Reports and Correspondence

Maidstone Osteopathic Clinic – Correspondence

British Naturopathic and Osteopathic Association – Public Relations Report (25/04/63) and Report of the International Relations Committee (25/04/63) Statement Board of Governors, British College of Naturopathy and Osteopathy (16/02/74)

Continued...

Society of Osteopaths News Bulletins
Journal of the Society of Osteopaths – Autumn 1976, Spring and Autumn 1977, Autumn 1978, Spring and Autumn 1981

A Hundred Years of Osteopathy in Great Britain by Thomas G Dummer and S G J Wernham

The Time Bomb under Alternative Medicine by Bob Bloomfield

Le Journal de l'Academie d'Ostéopathie, Janvier, 2000

Osteopathy in Britain The First Hundred Years by Dr Martin Collins, 2005

The Good Back Guide by Barrie Savory, 2006

Reports by Margery Bloomfield:-

An Outline Business Plan for the Move to Larger Premises

Public Relations/ Fundraising Campaign 18/12/96

Business Plan 12/07/96

International Academic Links and Activities 24/02/97